THE PREGNANT WOMAN'S COMFORT BOOK

A Self-Nurturing Guide to Your Emotional Well-Being During Pregnancy and Early Motherhood

JENNIFER LOUDEN

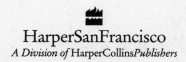

HarperSanFrancisco
A Division of HarperCollinsPublishers

To Lillian, my daughter

ALSO BY JENNIFER LOUDEN:

The Woman's Comfort Book
The Couple's Comfort Book
The Woman's Retreat Book
Comfort Secrets for Busy Women

THE PREGNANT WOMAN'S COMFORT BOOK: *A Self-Nurturing Guide to Your Emotional Well-Being During Pregnancy and Early Motherhood.* Copyright © 1995, 2004 by Jennifer Louden. All rights reserved. Printed in the United States of America. No part of this book may be used or reproduced in any manner whatsoever without written permission except in the case of brief quotations embodied in critical articles and reviews. For information address HarperCollins Publishers, 10 East 53rd Street, New York, NY 10022.

HarperCollins books may be purchased for educational, business, or sales promotional use. For information please write: Special Markets Department, HarperCollins Publishers, Inc., 10 East 53rd Street, New York, NY 10022.

HarperCollins Web site: http://www.harpercollins.com

HarperCollins®, ███ ®, and HarperSanFrancisco™ are trademarks of HarperCollins Publishers, Inc.

Library of Congress Cataloging-in-Publication Data
Louden, Jennifer.
    The pregnant woman's comfort book : a self-nurturing guide to your emotional
well-being during pregnancy and early motherhood / Jennifer Louden. — 1st ed.
        p. cm.
    Includes bibliographical references and index.
    ISBN 0–06–077672–2
    1. Pregnancy—Psychological aspects.   I. Title.
RG560.L68 1995
618.2'4—dc20   94–47638
                                                                                        CIP

05 06 07 08 09 RRD(H) 10 9 8 7 6 5 4 3 2 1

Contents

Foreword

This morning, my daughter asked me to help her put on her socks. Not because she couldn't put them on herself, but because her nail polish was wet.

Sigh. She is almost ten, most of her in childhood but a few toes groping toward tweendom.

When she snuggles against me now, and she snuggles only when she wants to, mostly when she is very tired or when we are watching a video, then I am blessed with the sweet drape of her dense body, a whiff of her fruity shampoo, the peach-like firmness of her calf against my hand. During these times I watch her, not the movie. I imprint her face on my memory. The line of her jaw, the freckles by her ear, the thick lashes that turn up just so.

If I could be where you are now, about to embark on motherhood, I would do things differently. That is so satisfying to declare in hindsight—how I would embrace my imperfections as a mother, how I would waste less energy wondering whether I was good enough, how I would listen to what I thought instead of what others told me about my child, how I would slow time down. Walk slower, eat slower, return fewer phone messages (no email back then!). How I would let the outside world engage in its mad dance without me.

Yeah, right.

Mothering is one of the most difficult emotional, spiritual, mental, and physical endeavors you will ever take on. It will flay you, lay your heart on your front doormat and stomp all over it. It will set you ablaze with such love you'll walk into the supermarket and want to hug everyone. It will also stab you with such anger you will walk into the supermarket and fantasize about running people over with your cart. It will stab you with the stark truth, a truth you will only be able to snatch a glance at and then quickly look away—that someday, this baby of yours is going to be hurt. Someday, this baby of yours is going to fail. Someday, far in the future, this grown-up baby of yours is going to die. And before that, you will. Meaning you will have to leave him or her.

I've heard it said that growing old is not for sissies. Well, neither is mothering. If you think for a moment you can get through this journey without being kind to yourself, if you think for a moment you can parent this child without learning to parent yourself, you're right. You can. Only, at the end of a year, or two, or twenty, you'll be the equivalent of the crushed litter of energy bars crumbs, colored pencil lead, and Northwest mud that lives in the backseat of my car.

Pluck and courage are very important self-care tools for any mother, as Ann Betz discovered, "I was four or five months pregnant, feeling tired, fat, and unattractive. Instead of the blissful time I was supposed to be having, pregnancy was bringing up all sorts of issues, my feelings about being a mother, my unresolved stuff with my own mom, and on and on. It was dammed uncomfortable. The books I was reading weren't helping a bit. Their tone was that I should A.) Do everything in my life thinking of the baby first, last, and only, and B.) I was carrying some sort of sacred burden for the whole community. I threw a couple of those books across the room. Where was the book that would help ME? Who would speak to me like the complicated adult I was? Then blessedly, someone gave me your book. This book understood that while I was carrying a baby, I was still me. It made me feel like I was normal to have worries and fears and eat too much sometimes and even at times (gasp) resent that I was carrying a baby and simply wanted what I wanted. That I could create my own experience and not fit myself into some 'Stepford Wife' ideal. Because of this shift, I was able to welcome my son into the world in a very different way. Once I was able to give myself permission to feel how I was feeling, we could be partners in the process. I was doing my job as best I could (being the imperfect—and normal—human being I am), and he was doing his job. Then after nine months, we met and fell in love."

Becoming a mother is about falling in love—with yourself, with your child, and on a good day, with your new role. Self-kindness brings countless precious gifts with it, not the least of which is the gift of being a better parent. A mother, a father, who loves herself or himself is a parent who can say no. A parent who gives herself permission to create her life is a parent who can look at her child and see that child, not her own unmet needs and ambitions. A parent who can speak to herself like the child she loves instead of like someone she loathes is a parent who can ask herself, "What does my child need? What do I need? How can everybody get a little of what they need today?"

Doing a good job of parenting means your child leaves. Creates his or her own life. You must have something of worth and value and depth left to create your own life from. It is a whole heck of a lot more difficult and painful to wait to create that value and depth when your child is ten or fifteen or twenty-five.

So lower your shoulders, curl up for a nap, and let yourself be the mother you will be. You will be enough. Truly.

Jennifer Louden
November 2003
Bainbridge Island, Washington

Introduction

Why Read This Book

You're pregnant and you want to be good to yourself. You want to glory in these moments, in your ability to foster life, but somehow you can't quite let yourself go. You feel guilty taking naps, slowing down, asking for help. You know you should relax and enjoy the attention your partner is giving you, take some time for yourself right now, stock up on sleep and sanity, but you just can't. There is so much to do. . . .

You and your partner have wanted a baby for so long. You're very happy, but sometimes you feel like there is an alien growing in your belly, taking over your life. People keep telling you how hard it is going to be after the baby is born, how little time you will have for yourself or your relationship. It's dawning on you that your life will never be the same, and you can't help but feel ambivalent about this baby, sometimes even angry and resentful.

You're exhausted. No, actually you feel like you've been run over by a UPS truck, lost all your ability to think or speak above a third grade level, and picking up your fork to bring it to your mouth makes you feel like you've just run a marathon. If this is what the next nine months, or even the next three, are going to feel like, you cringe at the thought of keeping up with your job, organizing the baby's room, picking a name, and the myriad of other details that must be taken care of, let alone doing anything enjoyable.

Now, what do you do?

A. Continue to live your life at the same pace, make yourself twice as uncomfortable and tired, and basically ignore your pregnancy until you're in labor?

B. Feel incredibly guilty that you have worries and doubts about being pregnant, then condemn yourself for being an inadequate mother while the baby's still in utero?

C. Sleep for nine months?

D. Sleep until he or she is in college?

E. Read *The Pregnant Woman's Comfort Book* and delight in your pregnancy as an amazing opportunity to learn the importance of self-nurturing and plant the roots of self-love so deep that when you become a mother, you will be able to replenish yourself and give authentically to your child without losing yourself?

Self-Care, Pregnancy, and Motherhood

It struck me the day after I found out I was pregnant. I was reaching for a fruit shake in the health food store. The usual debate was going on in my head: "You don't *need* to buy that. It's so expensive. You really don't deserve to buy that $2.49 drink for just *you*. You could make it more cheaply at home." Sometimes I argue with this insidious voice. Most days I lose. That day, I had no time for a struggle. A vibrant, new voice boomed through my head, "You are pregnant and you will have whatever you need. You will be good to yourself." I hastily searched the store to be sure no one else had heard this decree. And then I started to smile. A deeply delighted smile. Because it felt so good. Yes, I did deserve to be good to myself—not only because I was pregnant, but because I was alive! From that health food store epiphany, the idea was born that pregnancy is not something to be endured—a time of varicose veins and ridiculously frequent trips to the bathroom. Rather, it is a time of self-celebration, enriched inner life, and a chance to grasp that each woman not only richly deserves self-care but must have it if she is to survive and thrive as a mother. Pregnancy offers us the excuse to be gentle with ourselves. That excuse can become a habit. That habit can slowly become a lovingly held belief: "I *am* worth self-care, not just when I am carrying a child but every day."

Pregnancy is a time of upheaval, excitement, fear, ambivalence, unbridled joy, animal instinct, and love. The challenges of pregnancy seem perfectly designed to prepare us to be mothers. For example, getting up five times a night to pee correlates with getting up five times a night to feed. But there is another level to this preparation. The physical, emotional, and spiritual challenges of pregnancy can help us learn to love and accept ourselves, and that is the deeper preparation we need. By practicing healthy self-nurturing, we can discover a well-kept secret: that pregnancy is good for our bodies and our self-esteem. It can enhance our beauty, power, and strength. Pregnancy is an exquisite chance to taste the joyous freedom of self-love and self-celebration.

Pregnancy can make you fat, or it can allow you to appreciate the wonder of your body. Pregnancy can make you a raving lunatic, or it can give you clues from your raw emotions where you need to "cut to the chase," trim away the inconsequential. Pregnancy can make you extraordinarily exhausted, or it can give you cues to slow down and listen to your body, feed it what the baby and you need to thrive. I know pregnancy has many uncomfortable, even nasty, side effects. I'm not suggesting hemorrhoids have some magical potential for self-growth. I am suggesting that you can begin to learn to nurture yourself so that when faced with the physical rigors and cultural baggage of being a mother, you will be able to preserve a little bit of your self. Nurturing yourself becomes almost impossible when you are a mother—at the same time that it becomes even more important for your mental and physical health. (The one consistent underlying factor in postpartum depression seems to be an utter lack of nurturing, both from others and from the mother herself. Taking care of yourself now is the best insurance.) You can learn the essential skills of balancing your needs with those of your child's now, while you hug the toilet, when you are faced with having to ask for reassurance like never before, when you fantasize about quitting your job to be a full-time mom, when you cry because you are afraid of the momentous change shaking your life to its core.

But if all of this makes you indescribably weary, forget it. Use this book to have a more comfortable and enjoyable pregnancy. Doing this achieves the same thing.

Why I Wrote This Book

Believe it or not, becoming pregnant was not the reason I wrote this book. In fact, when my editor first suggested the idea, I rejected it. I felt my readers would think I was trying to turn every aspect of my life into a book. It didn't feel genuine. But as my pregnancy progressed and I began to struggle with everything from extraordinary exhaustion to troubling ambivalence to confusion about nutrition to an inability to ask for support, I started to see that the need to nurture and honor myself was intensified with the beginning of motherhood. Part of me was saying, "Yes! You deserve to be good to yourself!" and another part was moaning, "You're going to be a mother soon. Grow up. This self-nurturing stuff is ridiculous," while yet another part was chorusing, "You should take care of yourself only because of the baby. Anything extra just for you is silly, wasteful, and extravagant." This, coupled with the knowledge that I was having a daughter and desperately wanted to give her a legacy of self-love and self-respect, made me think there might be a need for a pregnancy comfort book.

I wrote this book not only because pregnancy is a physically uncomfortable time, but because it is an emotionally unnerving time. It is a spiritual explosion, a time of banging your head against the edict that women's *true* purpose is nurturing others. Dealing with the emotional and cultural conflicts was much more perplexing for me than surviving the leg cramps and ugly maternity clothes. The feeling of being connected to all of life was so wondrous, and yet nowhere did I find anyone talking about this. I felt a horrifying crush of guilt when I took a month to rest (I had little choice; I could do nothing else), but it was surpassed by the guilt I felt postpartum for not being able to handle hours of my baby crying without asking for help. The longing and sadness I felt as one chapter of my life ended also made me feel at fault. I was convinced that every other new mother was totally ecstatic.

I realized, with amazement, how both my discomfort *and* my joy were linked to self-nurturing: accepting myself even as I failed to be the perfect mother (in utero and beyond); making time each day for solitude and for listening to my inner voice; saying no and setting boundaries to help me spend my time in a nourishing, not depleting way;

giving myself healthy pleasure and fun; regularly connecting with and honoring the circle of life. This list makes self-nurturing sound pretty far-reaching. Becoming a mother has taught me that *self-nurturing* is in fact a code word for living an authentic life—something we as women have had to fight for the right to do. The pressure to be perfect mothers can drive us to give up our authentic selves by always serving others. I'm not suggesting that caring for children leads to becoming inauthentic persons. I am suggesting instead that equating motherhood with being completely self-sacrificing is what can rob us of our true selves. Becoming a mother does mean surrendering a lot of oneself to this new relationship, but it does not mean surrendering one's true self. It is precisely during motherhood that we need to nurture ourselves the most, for the sake of both our health and our children's well-being. Self-nurturing makes for a healthy mom.

What This Book Is Not About

There is a fine line between positing that pregnancy can be a time of accelerated inner learning and self-celebration, and making you feel like a failure if pregnancy is not a religious experience for you. Everybody is telling you to take it easy. To relax. To be good to yourself. It becomes a mandate, another reason to feel guilty about your lack of perfection. If you are not eating enough leafy green vegetables or doing your Kegel exercise one hundred times a day or playing Mozart for the fetus, you are already a bad mother. My goal is to make you emotionally more comfortable, to help you have a more pleasurable time, not to add another *should* to your life. Please, please, don't let the critical voices in your head stick this book in your face when you are feeling your most exhausted: "See! If you really wanted this baby and if you were really a competent woman who could handle being a mother, you would do everything in this book tonight. But of course, you can't. A failure again!" (Perhaps your critical voices aren't as nasty as mine.)

Please, take what you like, and throw the rest out the window—along with the idea that there is a right way to be pregnant or a right way to give birth or a right way to be a mother.

Every Pregnancy Is Unique

One thing I found annoying, confusing, and sometimes alarming was how most books on pregnancy divide the experience into trimesters. You will feel morning sickness at this time, be magically better on this date, then you will be incredibly horny starting at this time, and at the end you will feel like you have PMS and are wearing your tightest jeans on the muggiest day of the year. When my experience differed from what a book said was typical, I worried. I felt weird. So this book is not divided into trimesters, nor do I make any neat suppositions about when you will encounter what. Overwhelmingly, what my research taught me was *every woman's experience is completely different.* If there is one comforting mantra to repeat, it is: My pregnancy is unique. I am unique. My baby is unique.

You Need Other Women

It would be great if when we were pregnant we could go live, at least part of the time, with other pregnant women. Talking to someone who is going through the same experience you are or who has walked this road a few months before is incredibly comforting during pregnancy. You feel overwhelmed: the whole experience is so utterly unknown, ends with a possibly very painful bang, and then continues for the rest of your life. I offer this book to you in the spirit of one who has gone before and taken notes and then asked lots of other mothers for advice and taken their notes. This book won't replace the need for several friendly cohorts to compare expanding bellies with, but I hope it will help you survive, enjoy, and honor yourself as you prepare to be a mom.

How to Use This Book

This is a reference book for pregnancy. It is not meant to be read at one sitting or at one time in your pregnancy. There are lots of exercises and suggestions for self-growth in this book, along with ideas for making you more emotionally comfortable. Parts of the book at one time may seem absurd or not make sense or not interest you, but at another time they may be just the thing to help you feel better. Because you may feel so different in the third month than you do in the sixth, I have collected a wide range of suggestions and exercises. Use the chart in the middle of the book to help you locate what you need as your needs change.

You are participating in life's greatest mystery at the same time you prepare for the hardest job you will ever do. You deserve the very best now and after you become a mom. Be good to yourself and ask others to be good to you too.

Nurturing Yourself During Pregnancy

You'll Need:

Your journal or paper, and a pen.

Bubble baths, country music, historical novels, solitude—whatever makes you feel contented and cozy.

The courage to set limits and say no.

When to Do It:

- When you are worn to the bone but it would never occur to you to cancel your third cousin's visit from out of town or to miss the wedding of a colleague, or to leave work before 10 P.M.

- If your idea of being good to yourself involves tax receipts, Lean Cuisine, and reruns of *Punky Brewster*.

- When pregnancy has physically forced you to take it easy, but you can't relax because you feel too pressured by everything you should be doing.

- If creating an enjoyable, enriching, exceptional pregnancy sounds grand.

What Is It?

The kernel, the gist, the essence of nurturing yourself during pregnancy is treating yourself as if you were in the womb. Believing you have the right to be cared for by others, to be supported. Understanding how frightening and exhilarating it can be to open yourself to the new identity growing inside you: the identity of you as a mother. Grasping that you're in the midst of one of the biggest life transitions you will ever experience, and at the end of this transformation you are going to be called upon to do more giving than you ever have done and for an extended period of time (motherhood is about endurance). If you're not good to yourself now, if you don't take time to replenish and enjoy yourself, how are you going to do it after the baby arrives? For veteran moms, it is already difficult to find time for yourself. But it is going to be exponentially more difficult after you add your new baby to your life's equation. So although you feel you should be putting all your focus on helping your first child(ren) adjust, some time and attention must be given to you too.

If you don't fit the traditional picture of motherhood, your need for self-nurturing multiplies. Single, married but unsupported by your partner, lesbian, disabled, older: all of these realities can leave you feeling exposed and craving support. For example, strangers will ask about your pregnancy, always assuming you have a happy husband at home. When you don't, you may feel forced to explain, lie, or feel defensive. Older or disabled women may experience people judging them, in effect saying, "How dare you be pregnant!" Even when you are comfortable and happy with your choices, this can be wearying. Women who have struggled to become pregnant may feel "on-stage" or fragile. Women carrying twins have an increased need for nurturing. You all must take especially excellent care of yourself now because you face so much additional pressure.

For Whitney Kershaw, mother of Ian and Lily, pregnancy was the first time her life became her own. She has been a professional actress, dancer, and singer since she was eight, always being told what to do and always being asked, "So, what are you doing next?" With her first pregnancy, she felt, "Finally, I didn't have to prove myself, because it was obvious what I was doing. I became valuable for me, not for what show I'm doing, or what award I won." For Whitney, nurturing herself became her way of life. She gave herself the gift of spending most her pregnancy "doing everything I had never had the time for. *I finally believed I deserved to take care of myself.* Before I got pregnant, I didn't feel worthy. [This from a woman who has danced on Broadway and starred in a TV series—just so you know that beautiful, talented, accomplished women struggle with the belief they are not worth self-care.] My pregnancies were a peak time in my life because I went with my body rhythms, I did what I wanted, I felt wonderful because I was doing good things for me."

Jodie, mother of Livingston, reported a similar experience. "I made time three times a week to attend exercise class no matter how crazy work was. I would have never taken the time before. Pregnancy made me take better care of myself. I felt absolute clarity for perhaps the first time in my life. You *can* feel strong, healthy, and empowered. Every bit is so unique, you only have this one time. The most important thing is to be present."

I hope this chapter, this book, will help you create similarly wonderful, centered, playful, true-to-yourself feelings throughout pregnancy and motherhood.

What to Do:

What I Wish Someone Would Have Told Me

I wish someone had told me, when I was pregnant with my first baby, to take it easy. Loll in bed. Go to three movies in a row. Read lots of books. Do only what you want as much as possible. Celebrate your freedom. This may be your last time for many years (gulp). So repeat these phrases to yourself as often as possible: *Take it easy. Enjoy this time; it may never come again.* Write these words down and carry them in your purse or briefcase. It helps to be reminded.

See Fear.

Wrap your arms around the unknown. So many moms I interviewed said, "If I had only known what the whole thing was going to be like, especially labor, I could have relaxed. I wouldn't have been nearly as uptight, worried, afraid, ambivalent." (Take your pick.) I once led a group of women on a high ropes course (a series of balancing elements on ropes suspended forty to sixty feet in the air that you walk through wearing a harness attached to steel cables). Many of the participants felt fear, sometimes all-consuming, until they zipped down a pulley to the ground. Then they said, "That wasn't so hard. *If only I had known.*" Don't dismiss your fear, but remember: you have faced the unknown before. You can handle it.

See Forming Your Support Team.

Talk to other pregnant women *regularly.* It is a huge comfort. Find a pregnancy (and later mothering) mentor—a woman who has gone before you who can help you keep your perspective and perhaps your sense of humor. This can be particularly comforting for single moms and mothers trying to calculate the logistics of combining day care and work schedules.

Don't be afraid to ask for help. Don't hesitate to ask for help. Please, ask for help.

See How to Gracefully Ask for and Accept Support.

Work on believing you are a wonderful, unique, whole person. Motherhood is so fraught with guilt and doubt that shoring yourself up as much as possible now while you are pregnant helps a lot.

Remember there are many more suggestions in this book than time to do them. Do only what appeals and forget the rest!

Shouldn't I Focus on the Baby Instead of Myself?

While it is obvious that taking good care of the fetus growing inside of you is crucial, pregnancy isn't solely about the baby. It isn't only about birth either, although most of the attention is focused on labor. It is also about your becoming a mother, a fact that is overlooked or downplayed. If the baby and labor are your only concerns, you are set up to believe you don't matter and you will have little emotional preparation for the reality of being a mom. If you already have a hard time taking care of yourself (as most of us do), focusing only on the baby's wellbeing and ignoring your own will be doubly tempting. It is so incredibly easy and familiar to believe that nurturance is only for others.

Of course you want to keep your baby's welfare firmly in mind (so taking care of yourself precludes late-night slam dancing and Kamikaze chasers), yet it is vital for you also to emphasize your own needs and desires.

Define Your Needs

Pregnancy can be a very needy time, both psychologically and physically, and your needs can leave you feeling frightened and confused. If you can determine what you need, you can then pinpoint what comforting actions would meet those needs and provide some relief. Clarifying what you need also reinforces your sense of self, which during pregnancy can feel under siege because your psychological boundaries are enlarging and becoming permeable to include the presence in your belly. Finally, the more you can find ways to recognize and meet your needs now, the more likely you will be to do so after the birth.

You'll need your pen and journal, or paper, for this. Complete this sentence as many times as you can as quickly as you can:

To feel nurtured and taken care of during my pregnancy, I need . . .

Next, consider the following list of needs supplied by women in various stages of pregnancy as well as postbirth.

- The need to be physically safe.

- The need to know everything in the house is repaired and freshly painted.

- The need to nest: to buy new sheets, to have my partner help me keep the house clean.

- The need to be surrounded by beautiful things.

- The need to have help eating right.

- The need to sleep without feeling guilty or pressured.

- The need to feel financially solid and prepared.

- The need not to have to worry about money or talk about budgets.

- The need for reassurance that everything will be okay, no matter what.

- The need for reassurance that my mate is going to stay with me during delivery and after the birth.

- The need to know my husband loves me and still finds me attractive.

- The need not to do anything besides make it to work.

- The need to quit work and relax.

- The need to be touched, cuddled, massaged a lot.

- The need not to have sex.

- The need to have lots of sex.

- The need to have lots of sex in ways we have never tried before.

- The need to masturbate.

- The need not to drive the car.

- The need to have others drive safely.

- The need to feel crisp and attractive.

- The need to take multiple showers daily.

- The need to get all my work done before the birth.

- The need to play a lot in the month or so before birth, to go out to eat, see movies, read a novel all day Sunday without distraction.

- The need for someone to care for my daughter and give me time alone regularly.

- The need to go out into nature often and alone.

- The need to cry a lot without anyone worrying or making a fuss.

- The need to grieve the changes in my life.

- The need to grieve not being alone with my son ever again.

- The need to talk to many people about having a baby and how great it is.

- The need to be with my baby a lot.

Copy from this list any of the needs that strike a chord in you, adding these to the ones you already came up with. Take enough time to name all your needs. Don't panic if your list seems long. Don't despair if you feel alone, with no one to help you meet these needs. (There is always time for despair and panic later.)

Next, go through your list and consider how you can fulfill each need. For example, my list looked like this:

NEED	HOW CAN I MEET THIS NEED?	WHO CAN HELP ME?
I need help eating well	Read nutrition books	
	Go shopping with someone	Sara
	Ask friends to bring over high-protein meals	Randi, Deb, Zahra
	Make up list of meal plans and recipes when feeling well	Chris

If you feel overwhelmed by all your needs, investigate just two or three right now, the ones that feel most manageable. Some of your needs may be hard to meet, and if you are single or your mate doesn't support your pregnancy, you may feel it is easier to ignore your inner longings. But the attempt to pay attention to your needs is nurturing and empowering in itself. And it will help you to find other people to support you.

Postpartum

Consider doing this exercise again, after the baby is born. Try completing this sentence:

To feel nurtured and taken care of during the next three months, I need . . .

Then consider each need, focusing especially on how others can help you. Repeat every three months for a year.

Giving Yourself Permission to Be Good to Yourself

After you figure out what you need, the next step is allowing yourself to meet those needs and *enjoy* doing so. Eight weeks into her pregnancy and feeling horrible, Lynn hosted a baby shower on Saturday and a brunch for her in-laws on Sunday. "It would never have occurred to me or my husband to cancel. I was sitting at the table on Sunday feeling so ill and all I wanted to do was go lie down in the living room, but it took me forever to ask everyone if they would mind moving to the living room. Then I insisted everyone sit on the couch while I lay on the floor." Being pregnant grants you special privileges. The trick is letting yourself take advantage of them, use them. When they become second nature you can continue this healthy self-nurturing behavior forever.

Try reminding yourself this time will never come again. Of course, that is true for every day of your life, but the rareness of pregnancy brings that reality home. This is the only time you will be pregnant with this child. If you can't say no when you want to, or you burn with guilt over not maintaining the same pace at work, you miss the wonder of this time. Little by little, start facing the reality you can't be everything to everybody and still be there for your child and yourself.

When you are feeling conflicted or unable to relax, talk with the voice of your pregnancy. Many inner voices are available for you to dialogue with. You may be most familiar with your internal critical or judgmental voices. Pregnancy provides a unique inner voice, what I think of as the energy of life, which can calm you and remind you what is important. (This may sound wacky, but bear with me.) Find a few moments when you can relax alone with your journal and a pen. Close your eyes and concentrate on breathing deeply into your belly. Feel the breath going down into your belly. After a minute or two, pick up your pen and write whatever first occurs to you. It might be a question like "Why can't I relax?" or it could be simply "Hello." Now step back and let the energy of your pregnancy answer your question. Don't strain, just tune in. Dialogue with this voice. An example:

I'm so tense.

Breathe. Feel the life in you.

I feel so scattered. I want to relax, but then I get caught up in everything I need to do.

Come back to the life in you. Focus on the fact you are being creative even when you sleep.

I also feel like I have to make this time so perfect, so relaxing. That stresses me out too.

What do you want to do? Stop worrying about what others think would make your time special. Focus on yourself.

I do feel special.

You are as unique and wonderful as the baby inside you. Feel the life surging through you. Feel me.

I'm afraid to.

Do it a little at a time. Just a little. Breathe.

I'll try. This could be good.

See Preparing for Birth. Use this technique whenever you are feeling bored, stressed, or off-center or when you are hating your pregnancy. It also works well when you are envisioning the kind of birth you want and perhaps feel you don't deserve.

Finally, if you can't allow yourself to relax and be good to yourself, allow yourself to be good to your soon-to-be child. Motivate yourself with "My baby needs to relax" or "My baby needs me to be good to myself." After this practice is well established, transfer this caring behavior to yourself. Visualize how intimately connected you and the baby are. Grasp for the realization that at your core, you are as innocent and lovable as your tender, tiny baby. Feel in your heart that caring for and loving your baby cannot be separated from caring for and loving yourself.

Cut to the Chase

Many pregnant women and new mothers experience feelings of impatience and find themselves becoming brusque and irritable. While there are many reasons for this, including increased sensitivity to your feelings (and sleep deprivation for new moms), behind this impatience can lie a dawning realization of what is important in your life, what matters the most. Intolerance springs up for anything or anyone who doesn't "cut to the chase," because you just aren't interested in spending time and energy on things that don't matter.

If you feel this impulse, honor it. Build on it. Rather than using this irritable energy to bite your mate's head off for not getting baby insurance yet, try to explain why arranging the insurance is important to you. Or use your vexation to clue you in to what you need to let go of or downplay in importance. Ask yourself when you're irritable, "What could I change so I wouldn't feel this way?"

Wendy found during her pregnancy that she slowed down and concentrated on nurturing herself and her child. "I needed to get into the rhythm of my life more. I wanted to get back to the basics of life. I found myself buying organic produce, cooking again, not returning phone calls. If I didn't want to do it, I let it fall away. I didn't want to feel pressured." Many women report being drawn inside. Other moms regretted they had not let themselves slow down. If you continue on your present course, will you have any major regrets? What would you change? Let yourself go.

When you are faced with a situation in which you would usually say yes even though you want to scream no, say something like, "I would like to help you, but my energy level is too low because of my pregnancy." Or, "I'm giving all my energy to this little being inside of me, and I just don't have any energy left over right now. I have to say no." Or, "I need to say no because if I don't lie down within the next five minutes, I may spontaneously combust." Use your exhaustion to motivate you to carve out private time.

Ask yourself often, "If I don't do it, and it doesn't get done, does it matter?" Or make a list of everything you have to do, then cross off everything that you can possibly put off or avoid until tomorrow. Do only what is absolutely necessary. (This is an especially good trick for the first few months after the birth.)

Look for bodily reactions to clue you in to where your life may need stripping down. Susan realized her early pregnancy nausea had as much to do with her job stress as it did with her hormones. "I felt like crap all week, but on Saturday I spent the day relaxing with three good friends and I felt so much better. Sunday night I started to feel ill again. It was then I realized I had to start taking a more sanguine attitude about work. And I did. With the baby in my belly, it just didn't matter as much if some agent yelled at me. I still love my job and want to do a good one, but I started having perspective for the first time in my life." Susan fostered that perspective by asking herself often, "What is most important to me right now?" Also, when she found herself getting uptight, she would close her eyes and focus on the life growing inside her, visualizing her budding child.

Investigate the shoulds in your life. Every time you catch yourself saying or thinking, "I should do that," you have probably identified an area of your life you can let go of. Try changing the should into a could and see if that helps you see new possibilities and choices for streamlining your life. "I should go shopping for Jack's wedding present" becomes "I could go shopping for Jack's wedding present."

See Resources.

Cutting to the chase is really about having the courage to set limits and be firm when you do so. If this feels like an area you need to work on, check out some of the many excellent books on the subject.

If You Could . . .

Self-nurturing springs from doing what makes you feel good. But sometimes, in the flurry of responsibilities, we forget what makes us feel good. Explore the questions below by writing everything that comes into your head. Forget about reality for a moment. Or, if writing feels like too much effort, use the questions as a starting point for daydreaming.

- To really, *truly* enjoy your pregnancy, what would you like to do? (Examples: Take some time off work, buy several nice maternity outfits, eat lots of ice cream.)

- Are you doing it or will you do it? If not, why not? Is there any way you can truly enjoy your pregnancy even for five minutes today?

- When you contemplate the phrase "being good to myself during pregnancy," what occurs to you? (Examples: Being gentle with myself, screening out the world by not reading the newspaper, getting lots of attention, sleep, sleep, sleep.)

Use the answers to these questions to make a list of what you want to do to nurture yourself during your pregnancy. Glance at this list every few days to remind yourself of the possibilities. Add to it when new ideas occur to you. Push yourself to transcend limiting thoughts like "I work; only women who don't work could do that" or "I have kids so I can't." Please give yourself at least a few of the things you enjoy.

See What's Going to Happen to Me After the Baby Is Born?: Affirm Your Sense of Self for help adding to your nurturing list.

Postpartum

Consider the phrase "being good to myself postpartum." What occurs to you? Make a list and keep it handy for nap times and free hours when, not knowing what to do with yourself, you end up watching the baby sleep.

Zen and the Art of Peeing

Pregnancy presents even the busiest woman with built-in comfort time—ripe opportunities to weave relaxation into your life, tune in to your inner self, and give yourself tidbits of pleasure.

Try taking a mini relaxation break when you pee. Making relaxation a habit prepares you for labor, when knowing how to relax and get out of your own way can make a big difference. When you sit down to pee, consciously relax your shoulders and jaw. Close your eyes. Inhale deeply (unless you are in a stinky bathroom) and say silently to yourself a centering word, for example, *peace* (or *chocolate* or *orgasm* or whatever; the choice is yours). Then exhale through your mouth. Repeat until you are ready to vacate your throne.

When you take your prenatal vitamins, whisper an affirmation to yourself. Try "It is an honor for me to be a mother" or "I am a mother in my own unique way" or "I know I will go into labor when my body and my baby are most ready for a safe labor and birth."

When you feel your baby kick, take a moment to think of something you have done recently that you are proud of, and heartily congratulate yourself. Small accomplishments count as much as big. It doesn't have to be associated with your pregnancy. Getting a report written, refinishing a rocking chair, eating enough protein, remembering your sister-in-law's birthday: try to *unconditionally* compliment yourself.

When you exercise, take a moment to praise your body, especially if you feel fat, uncoordinated, or ill. Visualize the increased oxygen in your blood flowing to the placenta and being transferred to your developing baby. Remind yourself your body is keeping two beings healthy and alive. Congratulate yourself on getting active, even if you did only three leg lifts and then *had* to have some peanut brittle to keep your strength up. It still counts!

Before or after your prenatal health care appointments, do something special for yourself. It can be as trifling as sitting in the shade of a tree and eating frozen yogurt or as extravagant as buying a new maternity top and then getting a pedicure and spending two hours browsing in your favorite bookstore. If nothing occurs to you, use any time you spend waiting for your doctor or midwife to ask yourself, "What would make me feel really good right now?"

When one of the discomforts of pregnancy strikes, perhaps a burp of indigestion or a cramp of constipation, ask yourself, "When is the last time I did something nourishing for myself?" Turn the discomfort into a reminder to treat yourself great.

Resources:

Addiction to Perfection, by Marion Woodman (Canada Inner City Books, 1982). The classic Jungian study of how perfection kills women.

Blessed Expectations: Nine Months of Wonder, Reflection, & Sweet Anticipation, by Judy Ford (Conari, 1997). Emotional, spiritual, physical comfort for the ups and down of pregnancy.

Celebrating Motherhood: A Comforting Companion for Every Expecting Mother, by Andrea Alban Gosline (Conari Press/Red Wheel Weiser, 2002). A treasure trove of wise, nurturing advice in a gorgeous format.

Having Twins, by Elizabeth Noble (Mariner Books, 2003). Pregnancy and birth, especially carrying to term.

Healthy Pregnancy and Successful Childbirth, by Belleruth Naparstek. Inspires confidence and gratitude for the body; feelings of safety, relaxation, protection and support; sets the stage for labor and conection with the baby.

Meditations During Pregnancy, by Beth Wilson Saavedra (Workman, 2001). A treasure of honest insight and support.

The Woman's Comfort Book, by Jennifer Louden (HarperSanFrancisco, 1992). Section on setting limits and saying no.

The Courage to Be Yourself, by Sue Patton Thoele (Conari Press, 2001). A classic in learning to stop pleasing others.

Too Good for Her Own Good, by Claudia Bepko and Jo-Ann Krestan (Harper & Row, 1990). Excellent exploration of taking too much responsibility. Help for when you can't stop doing for others.

Where to Draw the Line How to Set Healthy Boundaries Every Day, by Anne Katherine (Simon & Schuster, 2000). By setting boundaries you protect your time and energy for the things that matter most!

Websites:

Pregnancy Today
http://www.pregnancytoday.com

Pregnancy & Baby
http://www.PregnancyAndBaby.com

Everything Pregnancy
http://www.PregnancySearch.com

A Pregnancy Journal

You'll Need:

Something to write in. Pregnancy was one of the only times in my life I was given a fancy book and then actually wrote in it. However, a journal can be odd pieces of paper gathered together in a folder, a sketch pad, a composition book, a girl's lock-and-key diary, or whatever you wish.

Pens, pencils, watercolors; a variety of appealing media of expression adds an element of delight to journaling.

A safe place to keep your journal.

When to Do It:

- When you are experiencing intense dreams, fantasies, fears, or feelings (what pregnant woman doesn't?).

- When you feel you are staying on the surface of this experience and you wish you could penetrate deeper into your psyche.

- When you feel a burst of creative energy and aren't sure what to do with it.

What Is It?

"In their purest sense, words not only describe reality and communicate ideas and feelings but also bring into being the hidden, invisible, or obscure," writes Deena Metzger in *Writing for Your Life*. Being pregnant can toss us into a swirl of feelings, dreams, and primeval fears like never before. Pregnancy is a time ripe with insight. But these insights can easily flit away without developing—staying fuzzy, fading away. Keeping a journal allows our inner sight to become tangible, flesh itself out. For example, I lie in bed and a realization about my relationship with my mother darts through my brain. I can notice it, maybe think about it for a few moments and most likely lose it or at least not learn all that I could, or I can grab my journal and write about it. The act of writing enlarges, clarifies, takes me deeper. It also allows me to create a document of a significant rite of passage, a reference point for future growth. "Writing makes a map, and there is something about a journey that begs to have its passages marked," writes Christina Baldwin in *Life's Companion*. We deserve to mark our passages.

But because pregnancy feels like a time you *should* be making a record, that in itself may make you not want to. The intense fatigue may make you say, "Keep a journal? You have got to be kidding me." I felt the same way. Christopher, my partner, bought me a beautiful journal right after we found out I was "with child." I didn't write in it until month five. I was in the "just being" stage of pregnancy, not the discerning, growing, in-touch-with-my-inner-world stage. Plus, I was unable to lift my head from the pillow for quite a while. Don't feel guilty if the very idea of writing debilitates you. A journal is *not* a diary. You certainly don't have to write every day or record how well you are doing eating your leafy green vegetables. Write if *you* want to, about what *you* want.

This chapter offers some tools for enlarging your understanding of the changes you are going through and for celebrating your experience. They are offered as suggestions only, jumping-off points for your own exploration. There is no right way to keep your journal or to enjoy your pregnancy.

What to Do:

Gaining a Handhold

How many times have you heard yourself saying or thinking, "I can't believe I'm pregnant!" Even a planned pregnancy leaves you humbled with the enormity, the sheer incomprehensibility, of the event. Friends who are parents ominously whisper, "Your life is going to change forever." You may feel as if you are approaching a cliff, and someone is going to run up behind and shove you off, and you have no idea when they will push you or how far you will fall. Exploring these feelings in writing can make this radical adventure a tad more conceivable.

Place your writing materials close by. Lie down with your hands on your belly and breathe deeply for a few minutes. Let your mind wander around the phrase "being pregnant." When a few thoughts are flying around in your mind, pick up your journal and write everything that occurs to you. Don't censor yourself because "mothers-to-be aren't supposed to feel this way." Next, free-associate with the question

"What would make this pregnancy more real for me?" Record these impressions too.

Read your list. Are there any actions you would like to take? For example, when I asked myself, "What would make this pregnancy more real for me?" I came up with: buying a maternity outfit, visiting a baby clothing store, and watching a birth video. Do something concrete to help you comprehend that the cells multiplying inside you will soon be your daughter or son.

Childbearing and Personal Growth

Write what comes to mind in response to the statement "Childbearing offers women great opportunity for personal growth and transformation." Do you think this is true? Or is it utter self-help bull? Does the idea intrigue you? If you could, how would you like to grow or transform yourself during this time? Write a paragraph or make a list.

See Ambivalence: Grieving the Changes.

Conversely, how would you like *not* to grow and *not* to transform? It is equally important to recognize what you are not willing or ready to change or what you hope will remain the same. Pregnancy is a time of such great change that sometimes it feels good to focus on what is not going to change—at least if you can help it. Even if you know a certain change is coming, like saving for college or becoming more patient, acknowledge now if you don't like it.

An Ongoing List

Inside the front or back cover or in a specific section of your journal, compose an ongoing list of everything you wish to remember about your pregnancy. This is a great tool to use when you are too tired or busy to write much. Create an index of words to trigger your memory and function like an album of emotional snapshots, later helping you recall the feelings and moments that matter. Nothing is too small or big to list. For example:

- First food cravings—turkey burgers, apples, and sweet pickles

- Very irritable—felt bad that I took it out on Mom and Dad

- Baby first moved on December 18th

- Had a powerful dream—saw the baby's face above me

- Questioned my mother about my delivery—loved how strong she was

- Started having heartburn

- Chris and I visited pediatrician—felt like parents for first time

Your History

Part of taking care of yourself during pregnancy can include reveling in *your* story, concentrating on you to strengthen your own sense of self.

What is your birth story? Gather all the details you can. Talk to everyone, starting with your mom, your dad, grandparents, siblings, aunts, uncles, anyone with a version to tell.

What five stories about your birth and childhood have been imprinted in stone—the ones that are retold on your birthday, at family get-togethers, on holidays? Make a brief list. My list:

- Mom in labor and a train on the tracks. Dad going crazy with worry. A joke that he wanted her to crawl under the moving train.

- When I waved at Dad from the bassinet in the hospital the night I was born.

- When I hemorrhaged after my tonsils were taken out and almost died.

- Running away from home (all the way to the end of the front lawn).

- Giving a speech at sixth grade graduation ceremony.

List ten moments in your life you are most proud of and wish to share with your child someday.

The stories we tell others about ourselves hold precious information about how we perceive ourselves. What stories do you tell someone you are just getting to know to help him or her know you better? What stories do you tell someone you want to be closer to and are testing to see if you will be accepted? What stories do you never, ever tell anyone? (These questions are from Deena Metzger's *Writing for Your Life*.)

See What's Going to Happen to Me After the Baby Is Born?

Ask the significant people in your life to tell you something they cherish about you, something they respect, and their favorite memory of a wonderful time with you. (Yes, this is difficult to do. You will feel egotistical and weird. Jump in and do it anyway. It is part of the process of learning to love yourself so you can love your baby even more.)

Life Pledge to Your Baby

Consider what you are willing to pledge to your child. What do you want to give him, teach her, offer, promise, vow? You might want to compose this with your partner or with a friend if you are single mom. Consider what values are most sacred to you and what you most wish to pass on. What do you want your child to receive from you? What is yours to give? What promises can you make that are within your power to keep? You might find yourself focusing on the negative: "I promise never to invade your privacy like my father did." Transform any negatives, nevers, and shoulds by reworking them into affirmative statements. For example, "I pledge to respect your privacy."

See A Baby and Mother Blessing Journey.

If you are planning a naming ceremony or christening, consider reading your pledge to your child and your loved ones. I read my pledge during a blessing ritual and later on Lillian's naming day.

Looking Forward

What are you most looking forward to about having this child? What are your fantasies of play, togetherness, enjoyment? For example, Chris and I were sitting in the car after lunch one day when it occurred to me, "Our child will get to see the *Wizard of Oz* for the first time!" I actually started crying at the thought of all the marvels we would get to share with this little human being. List your fantasies, what you imagine doing with your infant, baby, child, teenager. Don't worry about chronological order or money or if he or she will share your interests. This doesn't have to be about reality.

Resources:

Mother's Nature Pregnancy Journal, by Andrea Alban Gosline (Marcel Schurman, 2001). A gorgeous journal with helpful prompts.

Letters for Tomorrow: A Journal for Expectant Moms and Dads, by Robin Freeman Bernstein (Main Street Books, 1995). A guided journal to share with your partner.

SoulCollage An Intuitive Collage Process for Individuals and Groups, by Seena B. Frost (Hanford Mead Publishers, 2001)

Writing for Your Life, by Deena Metzger (HarperSanFrancisco, 1992). A brilliant book using writing as a way to explore and enlarge your inner world. Nothing specifically about pregnancy.

How to Gracefully Ask for and Accept Support

You'll Need:

A pen and some paper or your journal.

Relaxing music.

When to Do It:

- When you've just picked a fight with your partner for doing the dishes, going to the grocery, or otherwise helping you.

- If you find yourself denying your needs to the point of making yourself uncomfortable or exhausted or even hurting yourself.

- If you find yourself trying to act like you did before you were pregnant, without even a nod to the changes taking place in your body.

- If when someone helps you, you spend the next five minutes saying thank you and promising to make it up to him or her in the very near future.

What Is It?

Intimately wrapped up with the tempestuous mood swings of pregnancy is the sometimes overwhelming feeling of being dependent: feeling vulnerable, exposed, physically weak. Pregnancy brings with it the realization that we can't do this alone, that we aren't able to do everything we did before, at least not at the same pace. While this need for help and support has its up side (not having to clean the kitty litter box for nine months), many women find it infuriating. Frustrating. Even degrading. Why?

- We have fought hard for our independence. We don't like the connotation that we are any less capable than anyone else, especially a man.

- We have been taught to give to others, to nurture others. It can be acutely uncomfortable to ask someone to nurture us or to accept help when it is offered.

- The institution of motherhood is founded on the belief that to be a good mother we must be selfless and utterly giving at all times or else we are negligent and inadequate.

- Accepting help implies, "Something is wrong with me; I can't do it all." We secretly believe that healthy, together women don't need help. It's okay for someone else to ask, but not me.

- Receiving support can trigger our fears of intimacy, make us wonder what someone is going to want in return.

- It is less complicated, "cleaner" to go it alone.

- We may feel we don't have a choice. Our partner may be less than enthusiastic, we may be alone, our friends may be primarily childless, or our family may reject our pregnancy. There doesn't seem to be anybody to support us.

If there is, almost universally, one area that requires growth for most women during pregnancy and postpartum, it is allowing others to nurture us, to aid us, to baby us. We cannot nurture ourselves if we don't allow others to help us. Sure, you say, I know this. But do you really know it, on a bone-deep level? You, me, all pregnant women must acknowledge to ourselves that when we let ourselves receive, let others help and support us, we have more to give. And because the biggest giving of our lives is about to commence, doesn't it make sense to stock up on all the love, assistance, and attention we can? If we get used to embracing help now, we can receive it after the baby is here, when we will need it even more. I'm not implying pregnancy means we forfeit our responsibility to ourselves. In fact, pregnancy requires us to take on the most awesome responsibility of all. But it is crucial to include in our definition of responsibility relaxing, receiving, and letting go, as well as taking charge, being independent, and making decisions.

What to Do:

How to Gracefully Ask for Help

If asking for help makes you feel something is wrong with you, by all means, start small. Ask for a hug from your partner. Ask a co-worker to field one phone call. Say no to something small and truly distasteful.

Pick thoughtfully and carefully whom you ask for help. For instance, during my first trimester I suffered almost constantly from low blood sugar, complicated by very specific food cravings. I needed to eat often, but I rarely wanted to eat what was in the refrigerator. Another pregnant friend had been urging me to ask for help. One night on the phone, I screwed up my courage and asked an old friend who lived nearby to bring me some Thai food. She refused, leaving me feeling rather disgusted with myself and angry with her. But we talked for another moment and it hit me: her brother is in the hospital, her mother is living with her, recovering from an illness too, and she has been taking care of everyone. The last thing she needs is to take care of me. *Do* ask for support, but consider carefully whom to ask.

Be honest with yourself about your fears. For most of us, asking for something for ourselves is tantamount to delivering our baby on Oprah. But if we ignore our fears, we can sabotage ourselves. (For instance, when I asked my friend to help and she couldn't, I told myself, "See, nobody likes me. Poor pitiful me. I'll just shut up and suffer alone.") When you ask for help, tell the person you are asking how hard or scary it is for you. Or ask yourself, "What am I afraid of?" in the moment of asking.

Avoid apologizing for needing help. It makes the person you are asking uncomfortable and encourages the martyr syndrome. For example: "Oh, I'm so sorry that I have needs, that I exist, but if you could just please, please, please help me, I'll be forever in your debt."

Practice makes not perfection but an expanded comfort zone. Get in the habit of asking for support once a day.

How to Gracefully Accept Help

When someone offers to do something for you, take a deep breath before you say *anything*. Count to five as you breathe. Look into the person's eyes, smile, and say, "Thank you." That's all. "Thank you." Realize he or she is giving you a gift. Allow yourself to feel the warmth and generosity this person is offering you.

Be conscious of the voices in your head that are saying, "You don't deserve this." "You can do this for yourself, you're not an invalid." "Won't this lead to a total inability to do anything for yourself?" Listen to the voices politely and then silently tell them, "I deserve support. A miracle is happening in my body, and I will honor that miracle by allowing people to help me." It sometimes helps also to say to yourself, "I deserve support because I'm pregnant *and* because I'm a valuable, worthwhile person."

Imagine the person who is helping you is helping your unborn child. Feel the gratitude and rightness of this: how your child deserves everything good, deserves help and support. Then imagine spreading this feeling of being worthy throughout yourself. You can visualize this as light or a warm wave of approval radiating out from your baby's heart throughout your body. Or imagine a miniature version of you floating in your own womb, receiving the love and support of your mate as he or she feeds you, or your best friend as he or she buys you a chic pregnancy outfit, or a total stranger as he or she carries your bags for you. Let the gift in.

Repeat to yourself, "The more I receive, the more I am able to give."

Resources:

Comfort Secrets for Busy Women, by Jennifer Louden (Source Books, 2003). See the chapter on receiving.

The Complete Single Mother, by Andrea Engber and Leah Klungness (Adams Business Media, 2000). A bible for single mothers.

Forming Your
Support Team

You'll Need:

Courage to connect with new people.

Childbirth education class.

Prenatal exercise class and/or pregnancy support group.

Postpartum mom's group and/or parenting classes.

Your journal or paper, and a pen.

When to Do It:

- When you find out you are pregnant.

- If you've just moved to a new place (lots of pregnant people move).

- If many of your friends are single or childless.

- If you are a mom who doesn't fit the neat definition of normal.

What Is It?

An extended support team is essential to your mental health. New moms, loving friends, an understanding family, an obstetrician or midwife who understands the kind of birth you want, a responsive pediatrician, and new and experienced parents to ply with questions: if only each of us could be blessed with such exquisite support. Pregnancy offers the opportunity to create or strengthen your support system so that it is in place postpartum when you really need it: when you haven't slept in two weeks, haven't had a shower in three days, haven't sat down to dinner since who knows when. *It is of utmost importance that you put time and energy into creating a community now that can support you as a new mom later.* We all need help. We all deserve community.

The good news is being pregnant opens you in an astonishing way to making friends and meeting new people. I'll never forget the morning a former neighbor, who had always been rather cool, walked by me in the front yard with her two-week-old baby. We talked for a few minutes, and her whole demeanor changed when I said, "I'm four months pregnant." Suddenly, she was offering books and maternity clothes, chatting away! I was flattered but also a tad hurt. I felt I was suddenly interesting only because I was pregnant. (I have since learned that parenting is such an intensively wondrous and anxiety-causing adventure, you tend to grab support and validation wherever you can. Hence people who aren't in the vortex of parenting are often temporarily uninteresting.) I was also thrilled to find it so easy to connect with other women. This thrill of connection continued throughout pregnancy and intensified as a new mother.

We should raise our children in tribes; each of these intensely demanding creatures needs six to eight adults to keep it fed, clean, soothed, and stimulated. But few of us still have a tribe intact, so it is up to each of us to create one. And even if you do have a great tribe, your pregnancy can be further enhanced by professional support and the support of other pregnant women. This support is critical for single moms, lesbian moms, older moms—for any woman who feels a lack of support from a partner, family, or the traditional community.

What to Do:

Make a Wish List

In a perfect world, how do you see yourself being supported now *and* after you give birth? Relax in the tub or light a few candles in a favorite spot in your house, and with your journal or paper nearby, let yourself fantasize for few minutes about what you desire in a tribe, a web of supporters, a collection of people who support you honestly and lovingly. Forget about reality. If you could have whatever kind of aid, assistance, backup you wanted, what would you wish for? Karen's wish list went like this: "I would attend an excellent twice-a-week prenatal exercise class. We would talk for a half hour about what is happening in our lives and bodies, then exercise. I would make friends with three of the women; they would be funny, open, interested in the same things I am. Ken would like their husbands. We would form a baby-sitting co-op after the babies are three months old. Other support would include my mother, who would stop telling me what I'm doing wrong, and would visit for one week after the birth but stay in a hotel. My obstetrician would really answer my questions and try as much as possible to honor my desire to have a VBAC [vaginal birth after cesarean]. My sister, who has no children and has never taken an interest in Zoe [Karen's first child], would visit me after Mom is gone, also staying in a hotel, and take care of me and Zoe for another week. I would also have a parade of friends and co-workers bringing casseroles or pots of soup every day for three weeks. At two months, I would help form a new mom's group. Ken would be as wonderful as he was the first time."

You can see from Karen's wish list that everything is not possible. For example, her mother's behavior is unlikely to change overnight, and staying in a hotel might be financially unfeasible. Who knows if she can find an exercise class like the one she describes, let alone meet women she likes and has common interests with?

See the questions under Finding a Great Health Care Provider.

So is this exercise futile and stupid? No! If you take the time to discover what you want, you are *a lot* more likely to make something happen. After writing her wish list, Karen realized how strained and unhappy she had been when her mother visited after Zoe was born. She also realized her relationship with her mother was worse than she had been willing to face. She decided to read about how to communicate with her mother. She asked her mother to come two weeks after the birth, when Karen felt she would need the help more. She also found a neighbor who was going away and needed a house sitter, and her mother stayed there. Karen tried to reach out to her sister, but that wasn't as successful and the sister didn't come to visit. For her baby shower, Karen asked only for support gifts: she supplied a chart for people to fill out on what night they would bring food, and another for what day they would call and talk to her about something *besides* the baby (Karen knew from Zoe's birth that no one pays much attention to the mom afterward). She also found an exercise class, not exactly what she wanted, but she did meet a few women with whom she became friendly. What worked better was finding an already functioning baby-sitting co-op. Asking specific questions of her obstetrician helped her work out a slightly more comfortable relationship with him.

See Preparing
for Postpartum.

"My second pregnancy and birth was so much easier and I felt so nurtured because I took steps throughout my pregnancy to arrange things that way. I focused more on me, which was hard, since I had to juggle the needs of a two year old. It also made me angry sometimes. Why aren't mothers supported more in our culture? I can't emphasize enough how creating a better support system the second time around made my life *a lot* better."

Let your imagination go, then take time to sift through what you wrote. What actions are you willing to take? Small steps are best. Locate a prenatal exercise class and attend one session. The following week, find out about a new mom's group for now or after the birth. After attending your exercise class a few times, strike up a conversation with a woman who looks interesting. Set tiny goals and be open to serendipitous surprises. I have found that when you get clear about what you honestly want, you may be handed it on a silver platter.

Finding Other Pregnant Women and New Parents

You can find other pregnant women and new parents in both obvious and obscure ways. The obvious places to look include a prenatal exercise class (excellent because you can start early and develop relationships naturally); a childbirth education class (do some reading about the different methods before you choose your class); and a pregnancy support group. Look in your yellow pages, ask your health care provider, scan your local newspaper, ask any pregnant women you see on the street, query people in your church or synagogue. Don't be shy; you've got a great excuse to reach out. I had never met my neighbor, Julie, but one day I cornered her when she was walking Dylan, her five month old. We were talking about labor, sex, and mothering values in no time at all. A less obvious place to find new friends is your health care provider's waiting room (you might see the same people over and over again). Or ask your health care provider to give you names of other mothers who are due around the same time as you. You could also try walking in the park or playground; visiting children's story hour at your library (for second-time moms especially, but don't be afraid to go without a child); asking friends, co-workers, and service people, "I'm looking for some other pregnant women to talk

See Resources in Preparing
for Birth.

to. Do you know anyone?"; asking a therapist who specializes in pre-natal issues; placing an ad to start your own support group; or tacking up a note that says, "New mom with infant seeking same for support. Call . . ."

Setting up a pregnancy or new mom support group can be as simple as finding four or five women who will commit to meeting once a week or every other week. Each meeting, someone brings snacks (very important with a group of pregnant or lactating women!), and someone starts the discussion with a specific question. Examples include: How does your body feel this week? Have you had any birth dreams? What do you imagine your birth will be like? What is your greatest fear about becoming a mother? You can trade maternity clothes, expanding your limited wardrobe. You could do a creative project together. You can simply get together to kvetch and crow about parenting.

See The Poetic Side of Pregnancy for creative project ideas.

Postpartum

As you are meeting new people, or at least thinking about it, keep in the back of your mind what your needs will be postbaby. Will you need help with an older child? Most first-time moms have no idea where to find baby-sitters. Start collecting names now. Also, collect favors by doing baby-sitting yourself and helping out other moms postpartum. Every casserole you deliver now can become a casserole delivered to you postpartum. However, be aware that a mom you help three weeks before your due date is not likely to be able to help you in a month—which is not to say you shouldn't reach out anyway. Often, helping others now makes it easier to take in support later, even if it is from different people.

Getting Support from Your Family

Getting support from your family may be even harder than getting it from your friends because your new baby affects the whole family's balance. If you are a single mom or in a same-sex partnership, old family issues can (painfully) reawaken.

> When one member of the family has a baby, it is not only the beginning of one new life, but also the beginning of new stages of life for all involved. With birth comes the implicit promise of regeneration and rebirth, practically and symbolically. A new generation is born and the older generation is forced to move forward.

So writes Joyce Block in *Motherhood as Metamorphosis*. You and your partner are not the only ones being affected by the tidal wave of change a new baby brings. A baby can mean the chance for your parents to redo the past, to do the things they wish they had—the things they didn't have the money or time for—to pass on the wisdom they've since discovered. Siblings will react as well. "The arrival of the new baby often highlights preexisting conflicts within sibling relationships, but it also provides an opportunity to make amends and resolve these conflicts indirectly," continues Block. But, although getting help from family members can be complicated, reaching out and including your family does have great potential for healing and strengthening your relationships.

Divide a piece of paper into three columns. Make a list of family members you would like to ask for help in the first column. In the second column, list specifically what you would like that person to do for you (some ideas may have come up in doing the Wish List exercise above). Don't rule out people because they live far away. Support can be many things, including phone calls, prayers, and silly greeting cards. In the third column, record reactions you foresee occurring when you ask this family member for support. To do this, close your eyes and imagine yourself as this person. Ask yourself:

What does having this child represent to this person?

What feelings, memories, old wounds, pleasant associations might be brought up?

What expectations do I have?

Don't censor your reactions; record them all. When you are finished with each person, study what you've written. What patterns can you see? (If you have a perceptive spouse, sibling, or even a friend who

knows your family, you might ask that person to help you unravel
your notes.) For example, perhaps you would like to ask your mother
to stay for two weeks, yet when you reconsider you realize she doesn't
like babies and hates staying with anyone for more than thirty-six
hours. Or are you not asking your sister for anything because in the
past she has been such a flake? But when you think about it, it's been
three years since she got sober, found a job, and settled down. Maybe
it is time to include her in your life again. Don't ignore your expectations. Unrealistic expectations of how your family is going to react to
your pregnancy and your child can be huge stumbling blocks. Work
from your experience of how your parents make you feel *today*, not
how they might make you feel at some mythic time in the future. Having a baby can make miracles happen, and roles can shift, but expecting that to happen can be setting yourself up for disappointment.

*See Preparing for
Postpartum.*

Note: Even if you have a very loving, straightforward, healthy family,
it still pays to spend a few minutes considering how each person
might react to your child's birth.

Getting Less Support from Your Family:
Dealing with Intrusion

Most of us have had the experience of a family member who offers too
much help or offers help when we want to learn to do it alone or tries
to bulldoze us into doing things his or her way. Stacey had this encounter: "My sister said she wanted to come out to help. I said, great,
how about two weeks after the birth? She informed me she had
already bought her plane ticket and was coming next week. I felt
completely overwhelmed and unable to deal with her, being very
pregnant and emotional." Or you might have the experience that Rene
had of constantly being told at family get-togethers what to eat, what
not to eat, that she better stop exercising, had she purchased the
layette yet, blah, blah, blah.

You can probably surmise that most of these intrusions won't go away.
It is important to set boundaries with your family, the people with
whom it is hardest and yet most important. That doesn't mean you
should institute sweeping changes or ironclad policies. "Mom, we will

allow you to see our baby only on the third Sunday of months with the letter *S* in them" is not the idea. However, by reflecting on your rights and desires, and by deciding what your bottom line is ("I can take Mom calling every day with advice on what to eat, but I will not tolerate her making disparaging remarks about my choice of health care provider"), you can take a stand where necessary to keep your pregnancy and especially your postpartum period free of damaging, unacceptable intrusions.

Make it clear as early as possible what level of support and input you desire. For example, I told my mom early in my pregnancy that in the first few weeks postpartum, I wanted her to care for me and let me care for the baby. She blinked, images of her cuddling my newborn disappearing, but weeks later I heard her repeating my request to friends as her own. Because I was able to tell her what I needed gently and before it was an emotionally volatile issue, conflict was adverted. State *from the beginning,* "We don't know what we will need from you after the baby is born, but as soon as we do, we'll be sure to tell you."

Deal with unwanted advice by becoming a duck—let it run off your back. Practice saying, "Thanks for the input," and then biting your tongue. Learn not to engage when a family member starts pushing your buttons. Either change the subject or listen politely and say, "Thank you for sharing." Later, let off steam with your mate, a friend, or in your journal.

If someone in your family has a substance abuse problem, now is the time for you to get help. Attend an Al-Anon meeting. Read a book on alcoholic family patterns. Use as your motivation the reality that family patterns are passed on, generation to generation.

See Resources for books on alcoholic family patterns.

The central struggle with an intrusive family member is between your needs and his or her needs. This is the central struggle of parenting and of most relationships. When faced with a situation, like your mother wanting to be at your birth or your mother-in-law coming to visit for three weeks two days after the birth and wanting to stay in your one-bedroom apartment, honor what *you* need, desire, wish for. Start now, in whatever small ways you can, to express what you want clearly and lovingly. Know too that families are the most difficult places to set boundaries, so congratulate yourself profusely every time you do.

Consider your role in the intrusion. *This is not about blame.* Sit down with your journal and write for five minutes on the question "How can I change my relationship with _____?" and five minutes on "What am I getting out of _____ treating me this way?" Repeat this exercise for each person who is bugging you.

You shouldn't have to stand up to your partner's family as well. Avoid the trap of thinking all emotional matters for both families are your sole responsibility. Take a step back from doing all the emotional work, and see if your partner fills the void.

There is always forgiveness. When meddlesome relatives poke their heads into your pregnancy, close your eyes and imagine them at a pleasant time in the past, a time when you loved them and got along well. Or imagine them as young children, innocent and sweet.

Postpartum

*See Preparing
for Postpartum.*

It cannot be stressed enough how precious, fragile, and emotionally reckless the first few weeks of postpartum are. You want this time to be as relaxing as possible. You crave nurturing. You do not want to be fighting with your family or spending your precious energy worrying about pleasing or entertaining someone else. Keep that in mind!

If you can't get your family out of your hair, or you've tried and it didn't work, you will survive. Planning and boundary setting reside neatly in the world of self-help books, but in life they are always messy, imperfect processes. If your sister-in-law still comes for a visit even when you asked her not to, that's okay. Make her change diapers and do laundry while you nap.

Single and Childless Friends

Pregnancy and birth are hard on friendships. Some will fall by the wayside, new ones will be formed, and others will change forever. What happens to some of our prepregnancy friendships can be subtle.

A friend doesn't understand why you are too tired to go out at 7:30 on a Friday night. After the baby arrives, he or she might want to hear your labor story only once, not a dozen times. You feel miffed. You call less. You drift apart. Or you simply can't find much to talk about anymore. Some friendships probably need to wilt; as sad as it is to acknowledge, some friendships have a limited life span. It is the special friends you *want* to keep that you need to make an effort for.

The best course of action is: decide which friendships are most important and give your time and energy to them. This doesn't mean you have to cut everyone else out of your life, but child rearing does require careful use of your time. If you aren't sure who is most important to you or you aren't able to say no to invitations that aren't top priority, you may find yourself without enough time to spend with the people who matter most.

Set aside time with friends you cherish to discuss any worries you or they may have about how your relationship may change. Discuss how you will handle conflicts as they arise because of not having enough time, having to change plans at the last minute, or not returning phone calls promptly. Most of us aren't comfortable disagreeing with a friend. The new baby comes along, our friend feels slighted but it is too uncomfortable to say so, so the friendship withers away. Better to plan now how you might discuss hurt feelings later.

Having friends who aren't mothers can be a true sanity check. One mother of two said, "I would say to my friend, 'Talk to me about your exciting life.' It was a welcome switch from baby concerns." She also said, "Babies are sinkholes for friendships. If they haven't had one, they don't understand how your entire day can be taken up by one little creature. They say, 'But *all* you have to do is take care of the baby.' Ha!"

Resources:

Imagine a Woman in Love with Herself: Embracing Your Wisdom and Wholeness, by Patricia Reilly (Conari, 1999). A moving meditation on creating an inner vision of self-love.

Keys to Your Highest Potential, by Martha Howard, MD (Audio). A powerful combo of hypnosis, imagery, and affirmations to remove self-imposed blocks to success.

Loving What Is, by Byron Katie with Stephen Mitchell (Harmony Books, 2002). Learn how to use a process called "The Work" to transform negative feelings into a new reality.

The Art of Forgiveness, Lovingkindness, and Peace, by Jack Kornfield (Bantam, 2002). A collection of age-old teachings, modern stories, and time-honored practices for bringing healing, peace, and compassion into your daily life.

The Courage to Heal: A Guide for Women Survivors of Child Sexual Abuse, by Ellen Bass and Laura Davis (Perennial, 1994). I learned about self-nurturing from this classic.

Toxic People: Ten Ways of Dealing with People Who Make Your Life Miserable, by Lillian Glass (St. Martin's Press, 1997). Learn 30 different "toxic" personality types and how to deal more effectively with them, as well as identify your own toxic behavior patterns.

Websites:

International MOMS Club
www.momsclub.org

Mocha Moms – A support group for stay-at-home mothers of color
www.mochamoms.org

MOPS—Mothers of Preschoolers (non-denominational Christian support)
www.mops.org

Mothers & More: The Network for Sequencing Women (combining parenting and paid employment)
www.mothersandmore.org

National Organization of Mothers of Twins Club
www.nomotc.org

All About Moms
www.allaboutmoms.com

Mid-Life Mother
www.midlifemother.com

Single Mothers Sharing Houses
http://www.co-abode.com

Parent's Place
www.parentsplace.com

20ish Parents
www.20ishparents.com

Birth Waves
www.birthwaves.com

With Child
www.withchild.com

Arm's Reach
www.armsreach.com

Finding a Great
Health Care Provider

When to Do It:

- At the risk of being flippant, when you find out you are pregnant.

- If you just assumed you would use your best friend's doctor.

- If you are afraid of doctors or have had a less-than-happy experience in the past.

What Is It?

Choosing who is going to help you birth your baby is one of the most important decisions you make in your life and the life of your growing baby. Your health care provider's training, experience, and style will directly affect your birth experience. Too many women think even though their doctor has a 25 percent C-section rate, they will be the exception.

It can seem tedious, daunting, and a waste of precious energy to interview health care providers when your best friend loved her doctor or your mother swears home birth is the only way to go. By all means, gather information from the people in your life and follow your instincts about what is right for you, but avoid leaving this decision to the path of least resistance. It is very self-nurturing to insist you get the best care available—care that fits your personality and birth vision.

You'll Need:

Your journal or paper, and a pen.

Referrals from friends, family, or childbirth education instructors.

A little patience, energy, and time to interview prospective health care providers.

*See Preparing for Birth
for how to do this.*

What to Do:

Find Your Health Care Provider

First you need to determine what kind of birth you want.

To find the doctor or midwife for you, check with childbirth educators who are *not* affiliated with any hospital. They may keep files about doctors, such as evaluations written by their patients, or be willing to give you recommendations. Ask them why they recommend who they do. Childbirth educators often can refer you to pediatricians as well. Check your yellow pages to see if there is a birth resource center in your community. Ask your local La Leche League. Ask other women you respect who have given birth, especially women who have had a VBAC.

Interviewing doctors is uncomfortable for many women. Doctors are authority figures and often don't encourage questions. This should be your first "comfort indicator" regarding your prospective health care provider: How do you feel interviewing, or even setting up an interview with this person? Trust your instincts. Do you feel brushed off, hurried, or overcharged? Not a good sign. Please don't rule out midwives. They provide lower-cost care, spend an average of an hour with you per visit, and are covered by some insurance plans. Interview at least one midwife or visit a birth center. Consider Jodie's story: "The first two visits with my OB I felt as if I was being rushed and he had literally five minutes to spend with me. I was told that my pelvis was too small and I would probably end up having a C-section. I decided to get a second opinion from the nurse-midwifery practice. The first time I saw Mary, she spent an hour with me. She asked me about everything, really got to know me. My first doctor confused me with someone else. The midwives took the time to know my home situation, my personality. I even felt they knew the baby, knew everything that could affect the birth. It was such a gift. For me, the high point of my month, when my baby seemed most real, was my appointment with the midwives. To feel that your health care provider has no time for you is to be cheated out of something very precious. Women need to know there is loving, personal care out there." With the support of her midwives, Jodie was able to give birth to 10-pound, 4-ounce Livingston at home without so much as a tear. Her story isn't about perfection or heroism during birth (it was *very* hard) but about feeling deeply supported, cared for, and validated by her health care providers. Barbara received equally wonderful care from her OBs. Her doctors actually sit with women during labor (very rare), perform no routine episiotomies, and encourage alternative approaches to birth such as walking, eating lightly during labor, and birthing in water. Insist on a health care provider who cares.

Finding a supportive health care provider is extra important for single moms. Nancy reported, "My OB/GYN was my principal male support person. I cried after our last appointment because he was the main person I had shared this experience with." Of course, you want to rely on friends and family too, but when looking for your health care provider, keep in mind how important this relationship could be to you.

Explore your options. It will feel time consuming and you may feel overwhelmed and weary. That's normal. Take it slow. Read and let your mind wander first, then interview when you are feeling a tad more normal. Don't panic; having your first exam at eight to even ten weeks is fine, unless you have had a miscarriage, are on a fertility program, or have experienced other complications in the past.

What to talk about in an interview:

Start with a very brief statement about what your birth values are, what is most important to you. For example, you may prefer pain medicine, a muted, quiet room to deliver in, and "rooming in" (having the baby in your room with you, not in the nursery). Other possible questions for the health care provider:

- What hospital do you use? Are there any options like a birth center, home, or birthing suite?

- What is the likelihood that you would deliver my baby? (Especially important if the health care provider is in practice with other physicians or midwives.) Will I see all the partners in your practice?

- What kind of routine prep do you order?

- What is your percentage of episiotomies? (Ask percentages for accuracy.)

- What is your C-section percentage?

- What percentage of women in your practice have unmedicated births?

- What birthing positions do you suggest, and what positions will you deliver the baby in?

- Do you put the baby on the mother's chest immediately and let him or her nurse? Can the newborn exam be performed on my chest?

- What do you consider normal for weight gain during pregnancy?

- Do you view birth as a medical procedure or as a natural event?

- What is your philosophy of birth? (This one is hard to ask and can catch doctors off-guard. Therefore, it is a valuable question.)

Watch your body and listen to your gut during the conversation. How do you feel about this person? Can you imagine yourself talking openly about your fears? Sharing your portrait of an ideal birth? Questioning him or her if you don't agree or aren't sure of something? How willing is he or she to answer your questions, to spend time talking? As you learn more, you'll have more questions to ask, but these give you a place to start in comparing practitioners and also a sense of whether or not they share your birthing style.

If you already have a doctor or midwife, ask him or her these questions at your next appointment. If you are unsatisfied or uneasy about his or her answers, you might want to consider a switch or ask to talk to another doctor in the practice.

Things a supportive health care provider does:

- Helps you gauge your nutrition, pointing out how you could get more of whatever you may be lacking.

- Responds fully to your questions.

- Remembers you from one visit to the next.

- Talks to you like a grown, responsible adult.

- Listens with care to your vision of your birth and studies your birth plan.

Things a supportive health care provider does not do:

- Scold you about your weight gain.

- Put you on a weight-loss diet or prescribe diuretics.

- Make you feel you have ten minutes of his or her time and that's it.

- Answer your questions vaguely or with "That's nothing for you to worry about."

- Talk more directly to your husband or partner than to you.

- Throw your birth plan into your file without reading it.

Spend time and energy now to find a practitioner who makes you feel safe but doesn't rob you of an active role. The effort will be well worth it.

The Magic of a Birth Support Person

"The newest member of the childbirth team, the birth assistant, can bridge a multitude of gaps in the care of the laboring couple, bringing essential added support not only to the mother, but also to the primary health care provider (doctor or midwife), to the hospital staff, and especially the father," writes Mayri Sagady, a birth support person and childbirth educator. A birth support person, birth assistant, or doula is professionally trained to attend you from early labor until after the birth. She does *not* replace your partner (a common fear voiced by men). Instead, she takes the pressure off your partner so your partner can focus solely on you. It is too much to expect your mate to care for you every moment, to remember every tidbit learned in childbirth education class, and to otherwise perform perfectly in a situation he or she may never have encountered before.

What does a birth support person do? Everything from providing consistent care between nursing shifts to advocating for your rights, explaining procedures to you, running errands (getting warm blankets, fresh pillows, grape Popsicles), and reminding you to drink plenty of fluids and go to the bathroom frequently. She can also assist you in breast-feeding, can photograph the birth, help with siblings, and offer initial or extended support postpartum. A birth support person is like having an extra brain working for you—a brain experienced in childbirth and much less likely to panic or communicate fear to you during labor. She is especially valuable if complications arise, when you may be too tired or confused to know what you want.

See Resources.

Sadly, most insurance plans do not yet cover birth assistants, but if you can find the money, it may be the best money you spend, much more valuable than the perfect crib and matching changing table. It is especially important to consider a birth assistant if you are in a situation where you have little choice over your doctor or don't even know who your doctor will be. One study by pediatricians Marshall Klaus and John Kennell has found doulas can significantly reduce the length and complications of labor. Ask your health care provider, childbirth educator, or prenatal exercise instructor for a list of possible assistants. Interview to find one you feel comfortable with; ask for references and their educational background.

Finding a Good Pediatrician

In the last month or two before you give birth, you need to find a pediatrician you can rely on and one who reflects your values. Nothing is worse than having a newborn wake up with a high fever and not having anyone you feel good about calling. All the same places you searched for your health care provider are good places to find a pediatrician. However, because you neither know your parenting style nor your baby, you may find later you wish to shift pediatricians. This makes interviewing several not as necessary, but do meet whomever you are going to use before the birth and do ask your partner to accompany you. Visiting the pediatrician can be a great way to make your mate or birth partner feel included.

Questions to ask your pediatrician:

- Under what circumstances can I call you after hours?

- What should I do if I can't reach you in an emergency? Who is your backup?

- Is it possible to consult you over the phone? Do you have telephone hours?

- How do you feel about childhood vaccines?

- How do you feel about Erythromycin eyedrops as opposed to silver nitrate or using none at all? (Erythromycin is the gentle choice, but your pediatrician should be willing to wait two hours to administer the drops because it blurs the baby's vision.)

- How do you feel about vitamin K? (Children are born without vitamin K. It is administered immediately after birth to help your baby's blood clot. However, there is debate if vitamin K is safe or necessary.)

The most important thing is to know you can call when you need to. Going through agony over whether to call the pediatrician is unnecessary. You want a doctor who can give you clear outlines about when to call, who is easy to reach or has partners you trust, and who you feel will be reassuring to a child.

The second most important thing is a doctor who makes your husband or partner feel included. Asking him questions, urging him to be an equal participant—to voice his fears and concerns—can be invaluable in encouraging a man to get involved.

Resources:

A Good Birth, A Safe Birth: Choosing and Having the Childbirth Experience You Want, Third Revised Edition, by Diana Korte and Roberta Scaer (Harvard Common Press, 1992). Slanted strongly towards natural childbirth. Doesn't cover how to neogiate your way through managed care.

Birthing from Within: An Extra-Ordinary Guide to Childbirth Preparation, by Pam England (Partera Press, 1998). One of the best books on preparing for birth. Filled with exercises to contact your feelings and body.

Complete Book of Pregnancy and Childbirth, by Sheila Kitzinger (Knopf, 2004). Another bible of childbirth.

Gentle Birth Choices: A Guide to Making Informed Decisions About Birthing Centers, Birth Attendants, Water Birth, Home Birth, Hospital Birth, by Barbara Harper with photographs by Suzanne Arms (Inner Traditions, 1994). Focus on water births. Well-documented and researched.

Mothering the Mother: How a Doula Can Help You Have a Shorter, Easier, and Healthier Birth, by John Kennell, Marshall H. Klaus, and Phyllis H. Klaus (Perseus Publishing, 2002). The lowdown on birth support.

National Association of Childbearing Centers, 3123 Gottschall Road, Perkiomenvilla, PA 18074-9546. Phone 215-234-8068. Send one dollar and you will receive a comprehensive list of free-standing birth centers and guidelines on how to choose a center. Or visit http://www.birthcenters.org

Pregnancy Childbirth and the Newborn: The Complete Guide, by Penny Simkin (Meadowbrook, 1991). Very complete and non-judgmental.

The Thinking Woman's Guide to a Better Birth, by Henci Goer with illustrations by Rhonda Wheeler (Perigee, 1999). Excellent guidance on making the most informed choices for your birth experience.

Websites:

MidWifery Today
http://www.midwiferytoday.com

America College of Nurse Midwives
http://www.acnm.org

Birth Parnters—huge resource site
http://www.birthpartners.com

Association of Labor Assistants &
Childbirth Educators
P.O. Box 390436
Cambridge, MA 02139
(tel) 617–441–2500
http://www.alace.org

Doulas of North America
1–888–788-Dona
http://www.dona.org

American College of Obstetricians
and Gynecologists
http://www.acog.org

Childbirth Organization
http://www.childbirth.org

Twins World
http://www.twinsworld.com

I Am a Body Without a Brain

When to Do It:

- When you want to relax and enjoy your changing body.

- When you are sick of feeling scattered, stupid, and silly.

- If the idea of lying around and doing nothing makes your skin crawl.

What Is It?

There is a quality of pregnancy that carries with it the potential for great enjoyment and also for great annoyance. I affectionately dubbed it "I am a body without a brain" because of the devastating feeling that my brain had taken a hiatus without asking my permission and all that was left was this eating, sleeping, burping animal. Why this time is greatly annoying is obvious: You forget things. Your bodily needs rule your life. You don't want to go to work and have to think. You can't make simple decisions, like what to have for dinner or where to go on your birthday. You may feel like Judy Holiday in a thirties screwball comedy.

But where does *enjoyment* enter the picture? The pleasure comes from allowing yourself to luxuriate in the feeling of being in your body, of listening to and responding to your instincts, of allowing yourself to simply *be* for a change instead of having to do. Existing on this simple level can be quite a sensual experience, a return to the body wisdom of childhood, if we can turn off the negative voices and enjoy

You'll Need:

Nothing.

See Nurturing Yourself During Pregnancy and How to Gracefully Ask for and Accept Support.

ourselves. Reaching this place of being can bring us down to earth, out of the realm of striving intellect, and into a place where we can learn to cherish our flesh, which can replenish our souls.

What to Do:

Practical Advice (Works Equally Well Postpartum)

Slow down. You are growing a baby inside your belly *and* running your life. Something has to give—and it's usually the frenetic pace of your life. If you take things more slowly, you will forget less. Pause often throughout your day to ask yourself, "What am I forgetting?" and "What do I need to pay attention to?" (This last question is a great way to integrate your intuition.) Do this especially before you leave the office at the end of the day, before you leave your house, or whenever you are feeling scattered and rushed.

Buy lots of Post-it Notes and small writing pads. Scatter these throughout your life. When you think of something you need or want to do, write it down. (A friend of mine is convinced the only difference between geniuses and the rest of us is the geniuses get up in the middle of the night or step out of a warm shower to write down the great idea they just had.) On the sticky notes, post reminders to yourself. Everywhere. On the front door you can tack a note querying, "Iron off? Stereo off? Heater turned down?" On your car visor, "You are operating heavy machinery. Take your time."

Designate a sacrosanct place for important things. For example, your keys always, always go on the hook by the back door. The airline and theater tickets and other irreplaceable items always go in the right-hand desk drawer.

See It's Not All in Your Head: Exhaustion for restorative yoga poses.

When you are unable to concentrate at work or think creatively, try eating a high protein snack. Or take a brief nap. Or breathe deeply, saying silently to yourself, "Breathing in energy, breathing out fatigue." Or put your feet up. Or sniff eucalyptus, pine, or cedar essential oil. Or quit for the day. Or switch to a less demanding task.

If you have an older child, enforce a rest time. Set a timer for one hour and explain to your child that this is rest time for both of you.

He doesn't have to sleep during this time, but he does have to play quietly in his room. Every time he comes out of his room before the timer goes off, extra time is added. Use this time to *rest*.

To Be Instead of to Do, That Is the Quest

To be. To exist without striving, doing, or accomplishing.

> For the first time in her life she was able to allow her body to relax and open itself to whatever life would bring. She was able to give herself permission to play. Being became the exquisite beauty of plum blossoms in spring, the fragrance of wet grass, the crystal song of a robin at dawn.

So writes Marion Woodman in her brilliant book *Addiction to Perfection*. Being is visceral stillness, a body-centered "I am," a lack of feeling pressured, a lack of feeling like you have to do anything. "When a woman stops *doing* she must learn how to simply be. Being is not a luxury; it is a discipline," writes family therapist Maureen Murdock in *The Heroine's Journey*. "*Being* requires accepting oneself, staying within oneself and not *doing* to prove oneself," she adds. Learning to be is one of the great tasks we are faced with in the development of our feminine selves. We have learned how to do, do perfectly, do constantly, but we must go back and learn how to be, consciously. Being is elusive, impossible to describe, but delicious to experience.

But why should we want to just be? Because it offers us a chance to renew our souls, to experience authentic self-nurturing. Being allows us to experience ourselves apart from labels, jobs, and expectations, apart from who we are *supposed* to be, helping us to stay in touch with our true identity; being grants us a moment in our bodies instead of our intellects, healing for a brief moment the painful split between body and spirit.

Pregnancy presents an outstanding chance to feel what it is like not to justify our existence every moment of the day. "An inherent law of nature is at work; growth cannot be rushed, nature will unfold organically," writes photographer and author Georgianne Cowan in her essay "The Sacred Womb." We know that pregnancy cannot be rushed and that we do not control what is happening. We may be amazed that we don't have to *do* anything and yet the baby still grows. We can learn *through pregnancy* how to step off the gerbil wheel of endless accomplishing, helping, and nurturing and back into the sacred quiet of our own minds and hearts—a place many of us have not visited since childhood. The overwhelming loudness of our body's needs centers us and gets us out of our heads. We learn that our bodies are amazing things, not just "clothes hangers," as writes Ellen Sue Stern in *Expecting Change*.

We can nurture life. This awareness can help us exist in the extraordinarily liberating thought, "I am alive and that is enough."

For me, being came when I surrendered to feeling exhausted, sick, and unable to move out of bed, much less write. The only thing I wanted to do was lie in bed and stare for hours at a time at the pecan tree full of squirrels. I felt so guilty, so worthless, so sure that I would spend the next nine months this way. But when I was able to let go of the negative voices and trust that my body knew what it was doing, I fell into what I now call the "just being state." The just being state is characterized by the lack of needing to do anything and the lack of feeling guilty about anything. I settled into myself and existed. Later, when I was feeling better, this state was something I had to cultivate, but it was much easier than it had ever been before. I felt like my body and my growing baby wanted me to just be for a few minutes every day, to encourage a restful, renewing respite to overtake me as often as possible.

Here are some ideas for encouraging being:

Being is more a state of what you *aren't* doing than what you are. You aren't beating yourself up for not doing the laundry or filling out your expense sheet or reading a "how to be a better mother" book. You are not *trying* to keep your mind clear. You are not *trying* to breathe deeply. You may have experienced this state before, perhaps lying in bed on a Sunday. There is an absence of pushing, tension, agendas, goals.

*See Nurturing Yourself
During Pregnancy: Giving
Yourself Permission to Be
Good to Yourself.*

Work with the internal voices that tell you you must do something every moment or you are a lazy good-for-nothing and will never accomplish anything worthwhile again.

Keep telling yourself, "I am enough. I don't have to do anything to be." It might help to do what Maureen Murdock recommends. Take a piece of paper and make three columns lengthwise. In column one, write down something you did today, for example, yoga. In column two, write "I am satisfied." And in column three, "And that's enough!" Murdock suggests that although this exercise seems simplistic, after a month or so of doing it, you will forget you were "never enough."

I AM A BODY
WITHOUT A BRAIN

Work with your fears; work on your trust that everything will be okay.

See Fear.

This might sound perverse, but try to enjoy the fatigue, the hunger, the chorus of bodily needs. Consider focusing on the up side of these changes by noticing any positive repercussions in your life. Does your body's increased demand for rest provide you with precious time to unwind? Can you enjoy the feeling of balance that comes from healthy eating? Ease into your body awareness; enjoy it like a cat enjoys a good stretch. Notice if you feel more centered.

Seek out physical nurturing that feeds your newly enhanced senses. Kristina bought deluxe scented massage oils. Harriet refused to wear clothes that didn't feel good against her skin and later focused on buying maternity clothes for their feel and texture. Monica found in her third trimester that she had a deep need to visit the sculpture garden near her office, to run her hand over the sculptures and lean against the huge Henry Moore creations there. I bought myself a variety of wonderful body lotions and applied them lavishly and got several massages. Delighting your body gives you a moment to appreciate it, encouraging a positive body image, which in turn lowers the barriers between being and doing.

See Am I Fat and Ugly or
Round and Beautiful?:
Honoring Your Body for
related body worship ideas.

Encourage moments of stillness in your daily life. Take a shower by candlelight. Read a meditation in Being Home by Gunilla Norris. Locate a farmer's market or wholesale market, buy a mass of flowers, and arrange them while listening to Vivaldi's Flute Concerto in D. Watch the moon rise or set. If you live in a warm climate, take a daily moment to walk outside barefoot and note what is happening. Float in the ocean. These actions function as gateways, encouraging "beingness" to flourish.

Take advantage of the periods of stillness, of reflective serenity, that overtake you. These moments are available, if you will only allow yourself to settle into them. If you are afraid of getting lost in your quiet reverie, set a timer to call you back.

Finally, get out of your own way. Let go. Celebrate, cherish, sink into this blessed time, when rocking in a rocking chair can be more than enough. Nurture this ability to relax and just be. Record it in your bones so that after the baby arrives, you will still be able to capture this stillness and use it to recharge yourself and to teach your child that we are human beings, not human doings.

Postpartum

Allow yourself to be with your baby. Rock and nurse, stare at those butterfly-soft feet, feed and nap, nap and snuggle. Let the immense amazement, the astonishment, the wonder, soak you through, wash you clean. Just being with your new babe provides the spiritual sustenance to help you adjust to motherhood. These moments will sustain you if you let go and allow yourself to melt into them.

Resources:

It's a Parent: Songs for the Lighter Side of Pregnancy (CD or cassette), by Randy Bobish and Rebecca Kupka. A hilarious musical journey through pregnancy, childbirth, and new parenthood. Available at 1–888-YOU-BABY.

Mozart for Mothers-to-Be (Polygram Records, 1996) CD. Excellent selections to reduce stress and help your brain focus.

UltraSound—Music for the Unborn Child (RCA, 1993). Selections of Debussy for calmness.

Websites:

The Interactive Pregnancy Calendar
http://www.pregnancycalendar.com

Pregnancy and Parenting Humor
http://www.thelaboroflove.com

Am I Fat and Ugly
or Round and Beautiful?

When to Do It:

- Early in pregnancy, before you are "showing" but after you've "thickened."

- If your partner, friend, mother, father, brother, or anyone else makes a derogatory remark about the width of your derriere or the size of your meal.

- When you feel like a fat, undesirable, lumpy, gray, waddling, unsexual creature.

- If you sense positive changes stirring in your attitudes about your body and you want to help these changes along.

What Is It?

Pregnancy can trigger our most loathsome feelings about our body, sending us into incessant bouts of asking "How fat do I *really* look? Come on, be honest." We might hide at home because we are just positive everyone can hear our thighs rubbing together, or we might joke, "If my boobs get any bigger, I'll have to get them their own credit card." Or pregnancy can free us from the tyranny of beauty, allowing us to luxuriate in our life-filled bellies, our wrinkles plumping out from water retention, our fecund roundness. Or we can react both ways simultaneously. (For instance, I worshiped my round belly but shuddered at the sight of my dimpled thighs.)

There is hardly a woman alive today who doesn't all too painfully know the price of living in a society obsessed with adolescent

You'll Need:

Music you can move to.

standards of beauty: perpetually young, firm-breasted, thin-thighed women are *it*. Where do pregnant women fit? How can we gain twenty-five, thirty, forty, or more pounds (especially if you are carrying twins) without feeling horrible, ugly, unsightly? How can we transform the painful dislocation from our bodies into a joyful celebration or at least a peaceful truce?

A friend told me that during her first pregnancy a man complained to her, "Why are you doing this to your beautiful body?" Pregnancy is supposed to ruin your body, age you, leave you with sagging breasts and a permanently maternal potbelly. But some women experience pregnancy as the first time they can honestly love and appreciate their physical shape, especially after birth. Susie, mother of one, wrote me, "I like my body more now. I like its pregnant shape because there is no unreasonable ideal that a pregnant body must strive to emulate." Another woman said with amazement, "*My body actually knows how to grow this baby.* All these years I've been trying to figure out what my body could do well—because it doesn't do beauty or being looked at well at all. Now I know at least one thing my body does beautifully, and I'm intent on finding others!"

What if you consider the changes to your body as part of the ritual of becoming a mother, a physical record of your rite of passage? Instead of viewing stretch marks as horrible violations of your flesh, what if you see them as honor badges signaling your membership in the largest club of all? What if pregnancy is the event we have been waiting for to reenter our physical selves, a chance to reclaim groundedness and connectedness? What if pregnancy can enhance your body image?

If you already like your body (and not just as long as everyone says, "Why, I didn't even know you were pregnant!"), consider the ideas in this chapter as ways to expand having fun with your body.

What to Do:

A Few Thoughts to Contemplate

Tracey, a photographer and mother of Zav, spent six months of her pregnancy flat on her back, unable to keep anything down. She even-

tually went into the hospital for an IV. Her legs became so thin she had
to sleep with a pillow between them. "I realized afterward that the
extra ten pounds I had always carried prepregnancy was my protection, it was my life saver. Because I was heavier when I got pregnant,
I was able to nurture the baby more when I was so sick and lost so
much weight." Now Tracey views her body as perfect, solid, and built
to survive.

Denise, an actress and mother of Harry, began her pregnancy with
vaginal bleeding. She also began her pregnancy with a fear of getting
fat. "It was fear of what the baby would do to my body that compelled
me to exercise too soon after the bleeding stopped, and I started
bleeding again. I couldn't let go of the exercise." Denise's compulsion
to exercise ended up causing her to spend a lot more time in bed, but
eventually the process of carrying and then having her beautiful son
helped her accept her body instead of fight it.

You don't want to force yourself to gain weight, but if you are saying to
yourself, "I don't need to gain more than twenty pounds. My mom
only gained seventeen. The baby takes what it needs no matter what,"
it is time to adjust your thinking. Jettison the idea that thin is perfect.
Recognize your body knows what to do. Acknowledge the unsur-
passed beauty of a pregnant body. Overcome the nasty little voice that
might be saying right now, "This writer is full of feminist, new age,
touchy-feely crap. If you gain too much weight, you'll never lose it.
Don't listen to her." This isn't about gaining weight to "cushion the
baby." It is about making sure our culture's obsession with thinness
doesn't hurt you or your baby.

When people ask you how much you've gained, say, "Enough."

Consider burning your scale. Getting weighed at your prenatal
appointment is often enough.

Honoring Your Body

Buy or make a special oil or lotion for use during your pregnancy.
Find a scent that you absolutely love. Just this once, splurge. After
you bathe, drench yourself with this lovely smelling concoction and

*See Appendix: Herbs, Oils,
and Other Natural
Comforters for delicious
massage oil recipes.*

concentrate on noticing and appreciating the changes you are going through. Take a little extra time. Rub the lotion on your breasts. Say to yourself, "My breasts can nourish life." See your breasts not as objects to be valued for their size and shape but as fully functioning miracles. Caress your belly and admire how much you can stretch. Your uterus starts out about half the size of your fist and ends up increasing thirty- to fortyfold! Appreciate this fact. Rub your body all over and tell yourself, "My body knows how to give birth. I can do this!" Make sure you take a moment to caress the parts of your body not directly involved in making the baby and try to feel a moment of love for them too.

From Marilyn, mother of Molly: Take a picture once a month. Lie on your back and point the camera through your breasts. Take one with your hand in the picture, holding up the number of fingers for how many months you are, and take one with just the landscape of your belly peeking up.

Take some artistic photos of your burgeoning belly. Pose wearing a black turtleneck and tights. Sit naked, silhouetted against a picture window. Slip into your partner's blue jeans, half unbuttoned to show off your belly. Use a camera with a self-timer if you are too embarrassed to pose for your mate or a friend.

When you catch yourself moaning "I'm so fat" or "I'm gaining too much weight" or thinking "I'll never be attractive or sexual again," stop. Take a deep breath and remind yourself *gently* that your body has a larger mission. Visualize your baby in your uterus. Visually and emotionally connect your extra flesh or bigger breasts or stretch marks to that baby.

See I Am a Body Without a Brain for help on being.

When you are feeling completely overwhelmed, angry, or resentful of your body changes, either surrender *or* do something. Doing something could entail exercise (be careful not to exhaust yourself; exhaustion during pregnancy is not good for the baby and it can take you days to recuperate), putting away all the mirrors in your house, buying a new maternity outfit, dyeing or painting designs on an old maternity outfit, getting a massage from a person with whom you feel totally comfortable, or going swimming and relishing the feeling of weightlessness and grace. Surrender could entail saying to yourself, "This is how I look. This stage in my life will not last forever. I can fight it or I can live with it." Surrender can mean hugging yourself and breathing deeply. It can involve allowing yourself to take a long nap. It can mean relinquishing the image you are accustomed to seeing in your mirror and how you used to look in your clothes. Or listen to a relaxation tape and imagine your aversion to gaining weight disappearing with each exhalation.

Your Partner's Acceptance

Many women spoke to me about the importance of their partners accepting and finding pleasure in their new body. "It had a direct relationship to how I felt," said one woman. "I could tell he didn't like the added weight, although he loved my bigger breasts, and it made me very uncomfortable and sad." Susie said, "Throughout my pregnancy, my partner's constant support and attention helped me be emotionally comfortable with my weight gain." Mary acknowledged, "I needed to know Julie still found me cute." How to communicate with your partner about this touchy subject?

Don't automatically assume your lover doesn't find you attractive. Too often we are our own worst enemies when it comes to eliciting negative reinforcement. "You think I'm fat, don't you?" "No honey, I think you look beautiful." "Beautiful? Do you need your eyes checked? I will never, ever believe you in the future when you say I'm beautiful. How can I be beautiful when I've got to pick up my butt with both hands to walk across the room? Beautiful, ha!" After hearing enough of this, your partner may just start to believe you. Imagine your mate loves your body—truly loves it—and accept the support when offered.

Collect pictures of pregnant women (look in maternity and parenting magazines and photocopy from books). Make a collage and post it on the refrigerator. Add some pictures of flowers opening and perhaps images of ancient birthing statues (check museum shops for postcards and greeting cards). If your partner asks why, explain that you are learning to appreciate the female form in a new way. If he makes a negative comment, consider leaving him. (Just kidding.) A negative

See Receiving the Nurturing You Need from Your Partner Postpartum (and Giving a Little Too).

comment is a great place to open up a dialogue about the wonder of the female body. Perhaps a little discussion about what your body is going through (and will go through) might produce the appropriate awe. For instance, retorting with "Did you know in the Huichol culture there are famous yarn paintings of a father in the rafters with a rope around his testicles? Below, the mother pulls on the rope during her labor contractions so he can share her labor pain. Pass the mashed potatoes, please." Another, perhaps a tad more mature approach, is to ask him, "What do you fear most about my body changing?" or "What do you fear most about having this baby?" Often, a partner's ambivalence is directly linked to his or her fear of being ignored once the baby arrives or fear you will not be sexually available (which you won't, at least for a while). If you can get these fears out in the open, you may be able to come up with concrete ways to deal with the situation if it does occur. Planning a night away at a romantic bed and breakfast six months after the baby is born is one possibility. Another is setting up a half hour weekly ritual starting six weeks after birth of giving each other attention, away from and without talking about the baby.

Clearly express to your partner how important it is that he or she appreciate your body. Do this at a cozy, relaxed, even romantic moment. Be specific. "I need you to tell me I'm still attractive. Often." Or "I would like it if you would massage my back and belly at least once a week." Be clear on what you need and insist on it.

If the negative comments persist, get outside help from a therapist, your health care provider, or someone your mate respects. Your mate does not have to love your body, but acceptance and support are *mandatory*. If you are not getting the support you crave, don't give up. Don't sabotage yourself by saying, "That's just how it is. He doesn't really mean it." Your most inner self doesn't know that; it wants your added weight to be okay. It is better to get these feelings out in the open than to let them fester. This issue can become a big black hole that keeps expanding, sucking your love into it, even years later.

Tell your partner, "I would like you to enjoy my changing body. What would make it easier for you?" See if you can accommodate any ideas that come up, without betraying yourself.

Women in lesbian partnerships won't (hopefully) need to educate their partners about how amazing the female body is, but you may find your partner is afraid of the changes happening to your body because they could happen to her too. There *is* something terrifying about the uterus expanding forty times in size or your blood doubling in volume. Be aware that remarks like "How could you possibly be this huge?" or "Does it hurt? You look so uncomfortable" are probably signs of your partner's anxiety, not indications of her finding you unattractive. Acknowledge any fears on your behalf as a way to open up a discussion. Together learn what your body is doing. Focus on the positive aspects. Assuage her guilt by letting her clean the bathroom and serve you lovely snacks in bed.

Accept that almost anyone is going to have some misgivings about you not looking the same, especially if fitness or slimness was a big part of your life or your relationship. It doesn't mean your partner is a bad person, but it does mean you must give yourself even more strokes and that you must talk about it openly. It also helps to solicit lots of support from your friends, other mothers, and mothers-to-be.

Fertility Dance

This dance is a prelude, a movement warm-up, to get your creative and bodily juices flowing so you can create personal exercise that also can be a ceremony of bodily respect. It was inspired by an exercise class created by Fredda Spirka. This is not intended to be a rigid formula, so experiment.

Make some time for yourself when you want to exercise and also revel in your sexy, powerful body. You need loose clothes, enough room to move about freely, and music that begins slowly and softly, then becomes more rhythmic and dynamic. Or pick two different selections, one slow, one wild.

Begin by sitting down, spine erect. Take a few deep breaths. Visualize your spine, all the way from your tailbone to your skull. Imagine energy moving up and down your spine with each breath you take. Spend a few minutes checking in with your body, noting where you are tense, where your fatigue, if any, feels located, how you feel about your body in general. Slowly become aware. . . .

Draw your attention down, into your uterus. Picture the life pulsing there. Meditate for a few moments on the statement "Life grows through me and in me. I am creating a life." Breathe in those words. Wrap your heart around them. When you can feel the energy of these words, stretch your arms out to your sides, then stretch over your head while taking a deep breath, then exhale as you bring your hands together, palms pressing together. Bring your hands down in front of your torso, gently pressing together and down. Do this several times—inhale while lifting hands out and over your head, exhale while pushing your hands together and down in front of you.

Move into a squatting position, back flat, elbows inside your knees, if this is comfortable, otherwise, knees as wide apart as possible. Breathe deeply and feel the music in your pelvis. Feel your pelvis gently opening. Relax your throat. Feel your throat softening and widening. Imagine your birth canal doing the same. While stretching, meditate briefly on "Life springs easily from me."

Fold slowly down onto your hands and knees. Bring your chin to your chest and scoop your hips, slowly and gently curving your spine inward and down. Then reverse, bringing your chin up toward the ceiling, opening your chest, and straightening your back. Feel the music in your spine as you meditate on the thought "My lower back is supple and well supported." Repeat this as many times as it feels good, concentrating on getting a good scoop in your hips.

Still on your hands and knees, widen your knees and place your hands in front of you far enough away from your body that you can keep your elbows straight (but not locked) while rocking backward and forward. As you rock, keep your shoulders relaxed and hips loose. Meditate on the words "Tenderly nurturing my body is my first priority." Breathe.

Move to your hands and feet, then slowly roll up, keeping your hips tucked under and unrolling one vertebra at a time, while being sure to breathe! Lift your hands over your head and stretch, then hold your belly, bend your knees, and roll your hips in a wide, sensuous circle. Reflect on the statement "The cradle of life is within me." Reverse direction and roll the other way in wide, slow, sexy circles.

Now you are warmed up. Let yourself become the expression of the creative force, of life, of birth as you spin out a dance of life. Feel the music with your body instead of your brain. Use your hips. Imagine you are a sunflower growing toward the life-giving sun. Or an otter cavorting through the bracing, salty sea. Or a woman from prehistory dancing to tribal drums. Or a sidewinder snake undulating through the desert. Dance the words "Life grows through me and in me. I am creating a life." You are the source, you are the container, you are life, and life is you. Feel this in your bones. Move in a way that extols your strength—squatting, push-ups, deep, slow stretches. Join the millions of women throughout history who have rolled, swelled, embraced, pushed, crawled their way into birth. See their spirits around you. Copy their moves. *Dance!*

End by hugging yourself and appreciating your body with all the awareness and awe you can muster. Be sure to do a few stretches, especially for your calf muscles.

Reexperiencing Childhood Sensations

Find a place outdoors where you can be comfortably naked. The ultimate is a deserted beach or lake where you can also swim in the sun. Or sun in your own or a friend's backyard. If being naked is too much to handle or impossible, wear a bikini. Or walk around your house naked. Wherever you are, imagine yourself as a child and your skin as baby skin—innocent, fresh, wrapped in the sensual. Delight yourself by fanning yourself, tickling yourself with a feather, massaging your feet with lotion. Lose yourself in the sensual details—the wind on your skin or the feel of a soft rug against your back.

If you aren't too large and if your pregnancy permits it, play a physical childhood game. You can do this with your own children, your mate, best friends, or your prenatal exercise class. Hide-and-seek, Mother-may-I?, tag, jacks—any game that allows you to sink into the moment.

After you've been playing for a while, check in with your body and see how it feels. Alive? Tingling? Capable? What memories does this game bring up about your body as a child? If you can, take a few moments to journal about ways you could incorporate any good feelings about your childhood body into your pregnant body—more ways to feel grounded, in contact with your physical self, accepting of it. Even if you aren't feeling great, this can be a good exercise because it can remind you that you will feel good again and that your body is capable and beautiful, just like when you were a child. Also, it can get your mind off feeling ill. (Note: Do this exercise with caution if you experienced abuse as a child.)

Resources:

Bountiful, Beautiful, Blissful: Experience the Natural Power of Pregnancy and Birth with Kundalini Yoga and Meditation, by Gurmukh Khalsa (St. Martin's Press, 2003). A deeply spiritual approach to pregnancy.

Pregnancy Fitness, by *Fitness Magazine* (Three Rivers Press, 1999). Great overview with all your fitness questions answered.

Prenatal Yoga, by Colette Crawford, RN. (Video). Custom yoga routine for pregnant women for a safe, gentle and energizing prenatal practice. Excellent! Call 206–547–9882 or on-line at various websites.

Prenatal Yoga, by Shiva Rea (Video or DVD). A stretches and strength-building exercises that help increase energy and stamina, and develop concentration to assist during labor and delivery. Available widely.

Stepping Through Pregnancy, by Nancy Anderson (Video). Sixty minute very low-impact step aerobic work-out. Intermediate. Call 1–800–433–6769 or visit http://www.collagevideo.com

Websites:

Midlife Mothering
http://www.midlifemommies.com

Fitness Online
www.fitnessonline.com

Tumultuous, Turbulent Feelings

When to Do It:

- If you catch yourself about to smash someone's car because he or she stole your parking spot or otherwise messed with you.

- If you have suffered from a low-level depression and suddenly feel alive but raw.

- If you want to use this time of intense feelings to gain insight into a certain relationship, become more assertive, or to prepare yourself to be a more empathetic mother.

- If you just want to survive.

What Is It?

"The whole veneer of everyday life is ripped away," said Diane, mother of two, describing the emotional roller coaster of pregnancy. The intensity of our emotions during pregnancy can help us to go inside, to strip away the polite, fake, learned behavior of the internalized pleaser, to discard what is not us, what has become outmoded and unnecessary, to give birth to a clearer, more instinctual nature. Yet being emotionally raw and responsive can cause problems. At work, we are expected to be logical and rational, compartmentalizing our lives, or we are considered unprofessional. "Swallow your feelings and don't rock the boat" is the cultural message. The emotional gauntlet of pregnancy can demand *a lot:* to grow, you want to experience your feelings to the fullest and enjoy the aliveness but without exposing yourself to unwanted criticism, trouble at work, or damage at home.

You'll Need:

A strong role model.

Solitude.

A journal or paper, and pen.

I experienced the emotions of pregnancy as a time of clarity, aliveness, and occasional bouts of nastiness, especially at the very beginning and near the end, when hormonal levels were highest. Some women experience depression and the need to hibernate. Others find pregnancy acts like a truth serum, forcing them to be honest and stand up for themselves where they never could or would have before. Whatever your experience, don't reduce your feelings (or let anyone else reduce your feelings) to "just hormones." It is infuriating when a woman's reality is reduced to her biology. Heightened hormonal levels are not *making* you have feelings, they are making you more aware of them. And don't worry if you haven't been hit by a barrage of increased sensitivities; it doesn't make your pregnancy any less special. Take what you need from this chapter and discard the rest! Forget being overwhelmed. Remember: each pregnancy, each time, is totally unique!

What to Do:

Learning to Be with Feelings

We can't experience our feelings if we distract ourselves with TV or busyness or block the sensations by denying they have worth. It is possible to learn to be with your feelings during this sometimes emotionally raw time. Here are some suggestions:

Retreat. Create solitude for yourself. It can be immeasurably easier to be with the full range of feelings when you have no one else's to consider. If, when alone, you start to feel overwhelmed, reassure yourself that no one ever spontaneously combusted from intense emotions. Don't project yourself into the future; take one moment at a time.

When you would rather do your taxes or clean the grout around the tub then experience your feelings, repeat as your mantra, "It is okay to feel. It is perfectly normal. I don't have to fight my feelings. I don't have to censor them." I reassured myself this way after seeing the movie *The House of the Spirits*. In the bathroom after the movie (a common place for reflection during pregnancy), I felt I would be crushed under the weight of my feelings: anguish at the inevitability of being separated from Chris when we die, fear that the impending birth of our child would fracture our recent honeymoon happiness, sadness that the afternoon together was over, regret that I couldn't write a book as good as Isabel Allende's. I was overcome with the urge to eat a pound of Mrs. Field's cookies (my favorite way to avoid feeling), but I stopped. I took a deep breath and repeated the mantra. It worked.

Link your feelings to the being growing inside you, your impending motherhood, and to any children you already have. Consider how intense and unfettered baby's emotions are; they have no idea what they are feeling or how to control it. Let your intense moments help you to understand your soon-to-be-baby's emotional world.

Gather comfort ahead of time to tap into when you are irritable, deluged, cranky, or sad. If you have other children, develop a list of neighbors, friends, other mothers, and relatives who can relieve you for one or two hours of self-nurturing and solitude. If your children are old enough to leave alone in a child-proofed room while you relax in another part of the house, then introduce the idea of "Mommy time." ("Mommy needs play time too. We did what you wanted this morning, now Mommy gets to do what she wants this afternoon" is one way to broach the subject.) Create a sanctuary at home or near work where you can go to soothe yourself. Develop ten-minute retreats from your responsibilities and children. For example, light a candle while you take a shower and imagine the water washing away all your negativity, all your worry; or sit in your favorite chair and stare out the window, letting all your worries fly away.

See But Isn't Self-Nurturing Impossible with Infants and Toddlers? for more self-nurturing ideas when you already have kids.

See The Spiritual Sustenance of Pregnancy: Establish a Reminder for more about sanctuaries.

Finding Your True Self

Peeling away the false and outmoded in your life can be a life-changing perk of pregnancy. It can signal the beginning of your new identity. Marion Woodman writes about this process in *The Pregnant Virgin*:

> Sorting the seeds is a daily process of ruthless honesty that allows us grain by grain to discover our Being. The Latin verb esse means "to be"; thus in discovering our Being we are discovering our essence. . . . Again and again we have to say to ourselves: What was my feeling in that situation—*not* my emotions, my feeling? My emotions may support my feeling, but emotions

are affective responses determined by complexes, momentary reactions to an immediate situation. Feeling, on the other hand, *evaluates what something is worth to me.* What am I willing to put energy into? What is no longer of value to me? . . ."

(Italics are mine. Woodman is not writing about pregnancy as a physiological condition but as psychological rebirth.) Feelings are indicators of what is of value, of where you should be putting your time, and of where you shouldn't be. Feelings can be appreciated as clues to how we need to adjust, what we need to tend to, what we need to let go of, instead of irrational, pesky, inconvenient nuisances.

Stop *in the moment* of feeling and ask yourself:

- "What am I feeling?" Naming the feeling brings it into the conscious realm.

- "When did I start feeling this way?" Consider what may have triggered you. Sometimes nothing will occur to you. If that is the case, fine. Some feelings are free floating or caused by something too long ago or too painful for you to deal with right now.

- "If I was honest with myself, what would this emotion tell me?" Asking yourself this question does *not* mean you have to take action. It only means you are willing to know. I'm not suggesting sweeping changes in your life, I'm suggesting considering what your sensitivity is about and what it can tell you.

Keep notes of the emotional shifts you cycle through in the ten lunar months of your pregnancy so you can appreciate your growth. For example, before I became pregnant, my writing took place according to a strict pattern that I felt powerless to change. This pattern included writing only in the morning and not being able to return to my work if seriously interrupted. Yet by the end of my pregnancy, I noticed how much more flexible I had become; I could grab ten minutes of writing here, an hour there. This might sound like an inconsequential alteration, but it was monumental for me, and I attributed it to my emotional self maturing, becoming less rigid, a personal requirement for my becoming a mother. Whatever the changes, big or small, applaud your development.

Pregnancy can offer renewed energy and insight into old issues and relationship impasses. "Therapists speak enthusiastically about the rapid growth and insights of women when they are pregnant," note Baldwin and Richardson in *Pregnant Feelings.* You might want to consider short-term therapy to work on your relationship with your mother, your partner, or your image of yourself as a mother. You might want to read *The Drama of the Gifted Child* by Alice Miller; *Mother Daughter Revolution* by Debold, Wilson, and Malave; *The Pregnant Virgin* by Marion Woodman; or *Welcome Home* by Sandra Ingerman. Or spend an hour in the self-help section of a good bookstore, thinking about a part of yourself (only one aspect) that you would like to work on during this pregnancy. Journaling is invaluable for learning about yourself; pick one issue you feel isn't resolved in your life, and write about it every day for a week.

I'm Afraid of Hurting Myself or People with My Feelings

Many of us fear being destroyed by our feelings (especially if you read Sylvia Plath in high school) or we unnecessarily fear hurting others we care about. It is a fine line between squelching yourself to preserve the peace and controlling yourself within appropriate bounds.

Ask yourself before you open your mouth, "Will saying this promote long-term growth between me and this person?" or "What are my reasons for saying what I am about to say?" Use these questions with absolute personal honesty; otherwise they fall into self-serving manipulation. If later you find yourself defending yourself with statements like "I was just being honest" or "I was just expressing myself," you may want to check your motives for speaking out. When used with care, these questions give you the opportunity to create a conscious dialogue between your rational self and your emotional self, without denying either. That is the healthy balance we all want to achieve. Which is not to say it is easy!

When you are out in the world, especially the workplace, where feelings seem to have little place, adopt an attitude of observation. Observe your torrent of passions and hatreds without judgment, without guilt, but also without acting on them. Visualize your feelings as a river flowing by, which you watch from the bank. Visualize yourself as a serene Buddhist monk watching the stream of life gushing by.

Express in your journal everything you would like to tell people that you cannot. Or write letters to them that you can later destroy about all the lousy things your boss does, how angry you are at your sister for being ill, how much you doubt your partner's ability to parent. Don't hide from your observations; do keep them to yourself.

Treat yourself with as much respect and tenderness as you can muster.

A Mood Can Be Just a Mood

In case I sound like every emotion in pregnancy must be a cause for great personal growth, let me remind you (and myself) that sometimes a mood is caused by not eating enough protein or eating too many sugar doughnuts. It may also be simple, straightforward anger at a reckless driver or an inept salesclerk who appears to be on Valium. Or you might be continuing to do too much and not taking care of yourself (which this book will soon remedy), or maybe you're suffering the strain of trying to keep all your balls in the air. When a mood is just a mood, relax to inspiring music. Eat some cheese and crackers or a no-nitrate turkey dog on a whole wheat bun or some low-fat frozen yogurt with hot fudge. Laugh at yourself; crying over AT&T commercials *is* funny! Pull your comforter over your nose and sleep.

I'm Depressed

Depression during pregnancy is almost completely ignored. Even close friends may not want to hear that you don't fit the stereotype of the blissed-out woman patting her tummy. You can end up feeling alienated and doubly morose, wanting only to withdraw.

See Resources in Postbirth Nourishment: Surviving the Emotions for names of organizations.

Mild depression is experienced by many pregnant women. However, if your depression is scaring you because of its intensity, duration, or sudden onset, you need to speak up. If you are feeling suicidal, unable to work, or are considering terminating your pregnancy after deciding to keep the fetus, if you are unsupported by family or a mate, suffering from debilitating vomiting, are a victim of child abuse, have experienced postpartum depression with a previous pregnancy, or have a history of being depressed, *get help*. Tell your health care provider. If he or she dismisses your feelings, find an organization that will mother you and refer you to someone who understands the sometimes very intense conflicts and stresses that come with pregnancy. (While these organizations specialize in postpartum depression, they can help with depression during pregnancy too.)

You are not crazy. You are not a bad mother. You do not have to suffer in silence because you have conflicts or doubts about being a mother. Be aware that if you seek therapy, your therapist's role is not to make you feel guilty or put undue pressure on you to conform to the ideal of happy motherhood. His or her role is to help you cope, survive, and make decisions that are best for you. Getting help can be ultimate act of self-love.

"Pregnancy was a time to beat myself up. I actually had lower self-esteem. I felt like an old women who was disguising herself as a young woman. Who are you to be pregnant? I felt ashamed of my big belly," related a single mother who gave birth in her forties. Other women spoke about feeling too young, as if everyone was staring at them, wondering if they were married, if they "had had a life already." If this sounds familiar, you must work to believe you are a wonderful person who has made the right choice. Support groups exist for single moms, teen moms, lesbian moms, moms over forty. If you are too depressed to join a group, do everything you can to pamper yourself. Allow yourself to grieve. Check to be sure you are not mind-reading: Are you sure everyone thinks your pregnancy is so horrible? Check out your perceptions by asking yourself, "How do I know what others are thinking about me?" Or ask people you love and trust what they are feeling.

See Nurturing Yourself During Pregnancy; Ambivalence: Grieving the Changes; and I Want My Mommy for helpful suggestions.

Subtract guilt from the feelings that are getting you down. Avoid getting sucked into the mythology of the perfect mother. We all parent to the best of our ability, and that includes in utero. We all feel ambivalence and regret. Some doctors and therapists have posited that in the womb the fetus feels and knows everything the mother is feeling, including her unconscious feelings. I say, your baby-to-be is not Big Brother. He or she can't feel every emotion, can't see your conflicts or confusion and cluck its barely formed tongue. *You have a right to feel your emotions.* Your emotional well-being matters too. Once again, the bottom line applies: love and take care of yourself, and you will be doing the best for your baby.

Investigate your depression. Dialogue with it in your journal by writing the question "Depression, what would you like to tell me?" across the top of your page. Breathe for a few moments, waiting for an answer to occur to you. Use your nondominant hand (the hand you don't usually write with) to record what your depression has to tell you. Ask it whatever questions you would like. You may feel like you are making it all up. That's fine, keep going. Write until you feel a sense of completion. Let it go if nothing comes to you. Try again later.

Indulge yourself in as much healthy self-nurturing as you can. It can help prevent your depression from worsening postpartum.

If you are concerned that your depression may worsen postpartum, obtain information on postpartum depression help in your area before you give birth. Alert your partner or a friend that you may need help. Have that person read a little bit about postpartum depression so she or he can help. Keep the information you gather in your postpartum file.

See Appendix: Herbs, Oils, and Other Natural Comforters for homeopathic relief of depression.

See Postbirth Nourishment: Surviving and Thriving: More Help and Resources for organizations and books.

Resources:

Homeopathy for Pregnancy, Birth, and Your Baby's First Year, by Miranda Castro (St. Martin's Press, 1993). Homeopathy can help with turbulent emotions.

Shouldn't I Be Happy?: Emotional Problems of Pregnant and Postpartum Women, by Dr. Misri (Free Press, 2002). Excellent guidance for depression, anxiety, and other feelings that may be sending you for a loop.

Websites:

About Pregnancy – articles about emotions
http://www.childbirth.org/articles/pregnancy/emotions.html

Connecting with Your Partner

When to Do It:

- If you are fearful of your partner leaving you (a common feeling).

- When you hunger for attention and nurturing from your mate.

- If your partner's attitude is "I can give up Monday night football for two weeks, three weeks max, but by then, everything better be back to normal."

- When you want to reach out and reassure your partner.

What Is It?

Connecting with your partner is an indispensable part of nurturing yourself during pregnancy. If you are a single mother, finding surrogate partners or birth partners, often in the form of several different people, is crucial. You may crave support for the immense changes happening in your body and psyche, reassurance that you are still attractive and that life will continue after the birth, or a strong desire to share your fantasies and worries. Your relationship can become central to your well-being and to your image of yourself as a mother.

You might fear that having a child (or adding another to the family) will hurt your relationship. While this doesn't have to be true, it is imperative to prepare for the coming change. The couples who fare the best are the ones who share certain traits: they have adjusted their expectations; they have begun to surrender their individual goals and

You'll Need:

Time together to talk.

Activities you love doing together, like strolls through autumn leaves, staying in bed all day reading and drinking tea, ice fishing, visiting gallery openings, rocking on a porch swing in the twilight.

Courage and time to face your expectations of each other as parents.

think of themselves as a family; they have learned to handle stress without taking it out on each other; they continue to share common interests; they have accepted that their marriage or partnership will be different after the baby; they have found ways to communicate and fight constructively; and they are open to dealing with the associations to their own childhood that having a child stirs up. Before you get depressed, be clear that this is a laundry list for a perfect partnership. Nobody does all these things. Realize *this is a process*. It is not possible or necessary to baby-proof your relationship. However, you can use this time to address the issue of change. *Couples who refuse to acknowledge that life and their relationship will change, or who put their relationship on hold indefinitely, run into trouble.*

What to Do:

Make Time for Fun

Arrange time away, just the two of you, before the baby comes. The best time to plan these outings is usually in the second trimester. Put some of the focus on doing activities that you enjoyed together in the beginning of your relationship. Also, think about doing one or two things you've never had the chance to do and that will become very difficult after the baby arrives.

It is easy to say, "Sure, we will spend lots of romantic time together before the baby's here," but you may find the months slipping away faster than you thought possible. The rush of getting ready for the baby, often accompanied by one or both of you working additional hours because you want to secure your job, earn overtime, or are feeling the need to provide, can peel away the hours till B day. Put up a calendar where you can both see it, and try to do something together each weekend. You won't make it every weekend, but trying means you probably will half the time.

If you already have a child, you will be wanting to spend time with him or her, but don't neglect to do things as a couple too.

Collect Positive Stories of Partners as Parents

Kris and her husband feared losing their relationship. What they needed was "affirmative stories of how relationships evolved. What did *change* mean exactly? How would it be different? How did people manage?" Jackie found it "irritating that people would say 'It will be different' and when I tried to press them to explain, they would just say, 'You'll see.'" Look for couples who can talk honestly, descriptively, and (overall) positively about their experience as parents. You may have to search a little, but it isn't impossible to find people who will answer your questions.

But He Isn't as Excited as I Am: Reaching Out to Your Mate

Just when you need to share this experience the most, your mate withdraws. Starts working late. Your sex life dries up (if it hasn't already because of nausea or exhaustion). You resent his lack of attention and support, which just spirals the relationship further into the pits. "Expected and expecting to be delighted, strong, and free, he puts on an act while his worries and fears mount internally. Desperately wanting some of the solicitous concern directed toward his wife but unable to ask for it, he departs into an unapproachable exile, which makes him feel more excluded still," writes Brad Sachs in *Things Just Haven't Been the Same*. Like you, your husband or partner may be feeling intense emotions, but he has no support for doing so. You are allowed to be emotionally mercurial. He is supposed to be stoically supportive. He may use this stoicism to manage his own uncomfortable, intense feelings, withdrawing in confusion when he most needs to give you support *and* when he most needs to get it. This can be further complicated by your need to have your mate feel no conflict about your pregnancy, to be strong and certain so that it is safe for you to be worried and conflicted. Asking him "Why aren't you excited?" can push him even further away. Inside he may be saying, "I *am* excited. But I am also terrified, sad, unsure, and I don't think that's okay."

See Ambivalence: Grieving
the Changes for a couple
ritual; and Receiving the
Nurturing You Need from
Your Partner Postpartum
(and Giving a Little Too):
Sharing Your Doubts for
an exercise to help you talk
about your misgivings.

Sometimes in a close relationship, the lines between what you are feeling and what your mate is feeling can become blurred. It is important to look for the unique ways in which he is experiencing your pregnancy and to become aware of the feelings he might be struggling with.

Try talking to him about your own doubts about becoming a mother or being ambivalent about the sacrifices and changes parenthood requires. Gently ask him if he shares any of these feelings. Be aware, however, that the more he feels this way, the more he may feel "found out" when offered support. It may take a few attempts.

One study found men worry more about their partner's pregnancy than their partners do. Watch for worries about your physical well-being and take them for signs of involvement. This might help you to see his nagging you about what you eat as pleasing instead of wildly annoying. Take him to your appointments so he can ask questions of your health care provider.

Use events like filling out insurance papers with "father's name" or shopping for a crib or picking up hand-me-down clothes at your aunt's to spark a discussion of his feelings and reactions to becoming a father. Try simple questions like, "Looking at these baby clothes makes her so much more real to me. How does it make you feel?" to get the conversational ball rolling.

Do some early baby-proofing around your home. This is the sort of concrete preparation many men can get a handle on. Remove poisonous plants, put plastic corners on sharp edges, place protective plugs in unused electric sockets, and ask him to plan what else needs to be done when crawling is suddenly upon you.

If you choose to have an ultrasound, get a picture of your baby and post it on the refrigerator door where he can see it daily.

Picking a name is often a good way to connect with each other, learn about each other's families, and share your vision of your growing child. Visit a bookstore together and peruse the child care section for a name book. As you leaf through it trying out different names on each other, ask your mate why he likes certain names or what they remind him of. If he is passionate about naming your child after someone in his family, find out why. A note of caution: naming can sometimes become a power struggle. This is one of first areas where you must learn to work together and compromise. If you find yourself getting into a conflict, step back and ask each other, "How are we going to handle these differences when the child is here?"

Can you imagine a group of men getting together for a father's group? As men parent more, they suffer from the same doubts and isolation mothers do, coupled with the message that it still isn't okay for them to open up and ask for reassurance. Instead of or in addition to an all-women's event, have a friend host a couples' or parents' shower. Ask everyone to share their wishes for you and your mate as parents.

Help your mate meet other expecting or new fathers. A childbirth education class with an equal focus on expectant fathers would be perfect, but such classes are unfortunately rare. Sometimes just being around men who are going through the same experience, without having to talk much about it, helps relieve the feeling of isolation and stress.

Expectant partners often have more vivid dreams and recall them more easily. Get in the habit of asking, "What did you dream last night?" Listen without interrupting. Meditate on the symbols his dream offers. Allow them to inform your unconscious.

Introduce a nightly ritual of placing both your hands and your partner's hands on your belly while you each visualize your baby floating safely inside. Take turns speaking to him or her. You can tell him what you did today or confess to her how much you love your mate or offer him a prayer for his safe passage into the world or tell her good night and sweet dreams.

Look for articles and books about the challenges and needs of expectant fathers and leave them by the toilet, by his reading chair, in his briefcase, wherever he could privately read them. Don't ask him if he did.

See Resources.

Many men experience anxiety about how they will perform during labor. You may want to nurture your partner by introducing the idea of hiring a birth support person; by taking childbirth education classes

See Finding a Great Health Care Provider: The Magic of a Birth Support Person.

together; by telling him exactly what you hope he will do; and by reassuring him that his presence is the most important element.

If Your Partner Is a Woman

Being pregnant in a lesbian partnership brings with it some unique pressures. Worries over differences between you as the biological mother and your partner as the nonbiological parent can be slippery and hard to articulate (your partner may fear not being as important to the child, you may worry that your feelings will be more intense); the reality of being different from traditional families and apprehension about how your child will be treated; the legal quagmire of adoption by the nonbiological parent; annoying details such as not being able to insure your family at a family rate or on your work plan; and perhaps alarm concerning a custody suit from the sperm donor or father can leave you exhausted and fighting about anything from coming out at work to politics. But these same issues can help you strengthen your relationship and your new family.

One of the best things you can do for each other is to create your own extended community. Other lesbian and gay parents, single mothers, family that is supportive, friends who love you: a safety net to help you feel that you have someone to rely on besides each other can ease the pressure.

Watch to be sure that you don't chronically take out your anger at this unevolved world (or an unsupportive family or having to play it straight at work) on your partner.

Discuss your fears. Spend time musing on how you will fashion your own sense of family, your own unique rituals and traditions.

Sample some of the ideas in the previous section, anything that helps your partner feel a part of your pregnancy. Take a childbirth education class together—and be sure that your teacher is supportive of lesbian parents.

As always, stay conscious of your feelings and be willing to share them, even if it means bringing up an issue that seemed like it was settled long ago.

Examining Your Expectations

Early parenting and relationship conflicts can be averted or eased by examining and communicating your expectations on many different issues. You may be thinking your first few days together as a family will be spent alone, listening to classical music and cooing over the baby. Your partner may envision visitors streaming through, the phone ringing, packages arriving, and him or her as the proud, beaming parent. A disaster is in the making if you don't communicate *now*. It is vital that you communicate your expectations for each other as parents.

Use the questions below to cultivate several conversations. Curl up by a fire, lie out under the stars, or hold each other in bed while you take turns *gently* investigating each other's expectations. *Be honest;* don't say what you think you should but what you truly, secretly hope will happen.

- What is your vision of labor? How do you expect me to act during labor? How do you expect to feel right after the birth?

- What do you imagine our homecoming from the hospital or birth center to be like (or if you have a home birth, what happens when the midwives leave)?

- What is your visualization of what our baby will look like? Act like?

- During the time we are both off from work and home together, what do you imagine the days will look like? Do you imagine relaxing, warm, happy times or stressful, sleep-deprived hell, or somewhere in between? Who will do what?

- What kind of support do you envision receiving from others?

- What will "normal life" look like with our new baby? When do you expect life to be "back to normal"?

- What do you expect we will do if we have a difficult (colicky or wakeful), premature, or sick baby?

- How do you see yourself making time for me after the baby is born?

- How do you see yourself making time for yourself after the baby is born?

- What are your assumptions about working or not?

- If both of us are working, what do we expect to do when the baby gets sick?

- What are your expectations of yourself as a mother or father?

- What are your expectations of me as a mother or father?

Yes, this is a very overwhelming list of questions. Please don't try to answer them all at one sitting. Take them one at a time. Use them to prepare for the great change, to draw closer together, not to add pressure or tension. However, if these questions completely freak you out, perhaps you could (gently) ask yourself why. If your partner refuses to contemplate these situations, you need to ask why.

An alternative way to explore your expectations is to take turns completing the sentence: I expect you to _____ after the baby is born. Relax together and go back and forth quickly, without stopping the flow to comment. After you feel you've aired enough, discuss where you differ and how you can make tentative plans about bottom-line issues like who gets up in the middle of the night with a sick child. While it is true that you can have no idea how your new life will unfold, it doesn't mean you have to let it catch you completely unprepared.

How Will the Baby Affect Our Relationship?

There is a "conspiracy of silence" regarding the reality of having babies, particularly the tremendous strain it puts on relationships. Husbands have a tendency to feel left out, wives have a tendency to be overwhelmed and hormonally imbalanced, and babies have a tendency to be utterly self-absorbed and needy. "If you don't have a system for resolving disputes," notes Jill (a new mother), "that's not the time to get one. I wish we had had an understanding from the get-go that this was going to be stressful, even awful, but that it would be worth it and we would come through it."

This quote jumped out at me when reading Melinda Marshall's book, *Good Enough Mothers*. My first reaction, when I was pregnant, was, I hate reading that crap, and I hate listening to people whine about how tough it is to have kids. If it is so god-awful, why do people keep doing it? It will be different for us, I kept repeating. It can't be that bad. My second reaction, now that I have a baby, is, You have a duty to warn women. It will be different for each woman, *but different doesn't mean easy.* It might be uncomfortable to hear now, but it is so vital to adjust yourself, as much as possible, to the coming change in your relationship. *Having a baby means you will have tense times.* Having a baby exacerbates your present differences and brings every conflict into painfully sharp relief.

If you feel you don't fight constructively now or you have problems communicating, take a couple's workshop together. See a therapist or at least get the name of a good one to have on hand postpartum. Read a good book together before bed. The couple is the core of the family. Polish your skills *now!*

Prepare for the worst. I know, this sounds pessimistic and awful, but if you don't give some thought to colic, sleep deprivation, months without sex, grandparents intruding, and how you will juggle work and child(ren), you are in for a terribly rude awakening. That rude awakening on top of everything else can send you over the edge.

Together visit other couples, and *together* help with their child(ren). Ask them what they like least about parenting. Ask them what they enjoy the most.

Locate parenting role models by thinking about parents you have known (or heard about or read about) who parented in a way you admire. (This can be especially helpful for moms who don't fit the traditional mold.) Ask your partner to do the same. Share your insights, focusing on the qualities you might want to imitate, and why.

CONNECTING WITH
YOUR PARTNER

*See What's Going to
Happen to Me After the
Baby Is Born?: Exploring
Your Changing Identity
and do this exercise
together.*

Discuss what individual goals you will each have to surrender to become a family. Spending time and energy raising a child or children means you will have much less time and energy for other aspects of your lives. You don't have to streamline your life yet, but it is an excellent idea to pin down a few specific changes, like realizing you both won't be able to exercise after work every day or Saturday night poker with the girls might have to change or you might not be able to keep up your vegetable garden.

Sex

Your need for physical comforting does not go away when you become pregnant (although it can feel like it, especially in the beginning). Perhaps no other pregnancy issue is so fraught with miscommunication, so sensitive, and so embarrassing (except perhaps taking a little poo during labor). "What if we never have sex again?" "Will having sex hurt the baby?" "I feel so unmotherly because I'm so horny" and "I don't want to have sex because the baby is right in between us" are all common concerns. Almost all the pregnancy books address the issue of sex, and from them you can learn that it is safe, men often do feel conflicted, and you may not want to do it at all. But what we are concerned with here is how sex can nurture you, can help you feel better about yourself as you make the transition into motherhood.

Make a list in answer to the question "How could my physical relationship with my partner make me feel better during my pregnancy?" Be selfish for a moment; *don't* consider your partner's needs. Share the items on your list with your partner at a mutually relaxing, private time. If necessary, experiment with asking for something you are concerned he or she won't want to give you. Your partner won't be able to meet all your needs, but asking will help you feel taken care of.

*See questions under
Expectations for help on
sorting out your idea of
what a mother is.*

If you don't feel like having sex, consider why—not because you have to change anything, not because you are wrong, but so you won't feel guilty and conflicted. Are you just too exhausted or sick? Fine. (However, one woman recounted that the only thing that relieved her nausea was sex.) Do you feel that mothers don't have sex? If so, it might be a good idea to explore your idea of what a mother is, both alone and with your mate. Do you feel unattractive? Many women do. If your partner was more supportive of your changing body, would you perhaps feel different? Are you worried that the baby senses you having sex and that is wrong? Perhaps thinking about how sex was treated in your home as you were growing up would be worthwhile. Or have a conversation with your mate about how you both plan to maintain your sexual identities once the baby is in the house.

CONNECTING WITH
YOUR PARTNER

See What's Going to
Happen to Me After the
Baby Is Born?: The Myth
of the Perfect Mother.

If sex is leaving you cold, don't neglect to explain how you are feeling to your mate and *don't stop touching.* Rhonda reported needing massage for relaxation and reassurance instead of pressure to have sex. She could verbalize this in a nonthreatening way to her mate. Unfortunately, rarely will your need to have less or no sex coincide with your mate's. Often, when one partner doesn't want to have sex and the other does, all touch is labeled as a precursor to sex and so becomes suspect. If you feel this may be an issue, see if you can agree not to have sex for two weeks (or a week or your first trimester—the amount of time is up to you). During that time, touch each other *a lot,* knowing it will not lead to sex, so no one will be disappointed and no one will feel pressured. Women in same-sex partnerships may find this to be less of an issue because touch is often a more central part of sex.

An inability to have an orgasm can leave you feeling awful. One study found that one out of four women were less likely to achieve orgasm regularly during pregnancy, especially during the last trimester. This may have something to do with the increased blood flow to your genitals. Whatever the reason, relax. You aren't passionless. You may still enjoy having sex if you don't feel the pressure to climax and if your mate doesn't feel any pressure to bring you to orgasm. Some women find they enjoy pleasuring their mates as a way to stay close but would rather receive hugs and backrubs in return.

If you want to make love a lot, you aren't alone either. Many women report feeling more aroused than ever and having better orgasms during pregnancy. Some women experience their first orgasms. One woman told me she had orgasms with her whole body! Several others found they wanted to masturbate frequently. This, combined with the experience of sex as a profound way to celebrate your creative relationship with your mate—after all, sex *was* how you created the life within you—can have you bopping away. Relish this heat!

*See Am I Fat and Ugly or
Round and Beautiful?:
Your Partner's Acceptance
for help.*

Insensitive remarks about your size or weight gain can do more to squelch your sex life than anything. If this is a problem, some exercises around acceptance might benefit both of you.

Be aware of your partner's conflicts about sex. Perhaps your mate is unsure about supporting you and the baby financially; this issue can have a tremendous effect on his desire to have sex. So can his fear of hurting the baby. Reassure him that during a normal pregnancy, the fetus is very well protected and sex will cause no harm. If you feel the pressure "to provide" is robbing your lover's libido, face it head-on outside the bedroom. Tell each other your worst fears. Share your grief over your life changing. Joke about what it will be like to be a lover and a mother. Reassure your mate that he will still be number one in your heart.

Getting Comfort for Your Fears from Your Mate

Incubating a baby can present you with an astounding array of life fears. Sharing these fears with your mate can make you feel better, but only if he or she can hear you without trying to fix things. The truth is, many of your worries *are* real. Confronting them and learning to live with them is part of the task of being a parent. When you are not beset with dread and anxiety, tell your lover to forget trying to talk you out of your worries. What you need is to be simply listened to, without being judged crazy or being offered solutions. Your mate can reassure you, hug you, rub your back, share worries, but if he or she tries to fix things, you will end up feeling not listened to.

If, however, you become so filled with anxiety and worry you can't sleep or function, you need to ask your partner to intercede. Fear can be paralyzing. If you are able, tell your lover what can be done: call a therapist, put up signs around the house that say "Don't worry because I love you," go through each fear with you and discuss what you can do to prevent it, hold you and whisper "Everything is going to be all right." Even if you don't know exactly what would help, *reach out.* Don't suffer alone.

Dependence and Interdependence

One of the central shifts that takes place when you become parents is a readjustment of your individuality, your dependence, and your interdependence. A common mistake is to think that by allowing yourself to depend more on your mate your individuality will be forfeited. This often gets carried over into the relationship: if you have a child, you lose your identity as a couple. This is not true. At least, it doesn't have to be.

When you feel dependent and vulnerable, take the risk of describing how you feel to your mate. Voice your fears about feeling this way. Ask your mate how your increased dependency makes him feel.

If dependency is difficult for you (as it is for many women), try this experiment. Set aside several hours in which you allow yourself to be very dependent on your partner. Go out to lunch and have your partner order your meal. Or go totally limp and let your partner move your body around. Have your sweetie give you a bath. Why do this? Because learning to be passive can be very helpful during birth (relaxing with the contractions). More important, learning to depend on your partner means you can avoid becoming Superparent, the all-knowing one who must do everything for the child and whose way is the only way.

See Receiving the Nurturing You Need from Your Partner Postpartum (and Giving a Little Too): Gatekeeping.

Together, decide on some ways you can maintain your coupleness *after* baby arrives. *Don't* wait to do this until after the birth. Make a list of things you enjoy doing together, keeping in mind how your time, freedom, and resources will be restricted. Keep this list handy so you don't find it crumpled under the take-out menus two years after the baby arrives.

Make a point of asking each other often, "What can I do to support you during this pregnancy?" The simple act of asking reminds you that during this time, each of you has special needs that the other can meet.

Acknowledge how your interdependence makes your family possible. For example, the way he cooks combines with the way you create a lovely home. She balances the checkbook, but you remember to write the mortgage or rent check on time. The way you plan ahead and remember details is coupled with the way he stays in the moment and helps you relax.

Resources:

Becoming Parents: How to Strengthen Your Marriage as Your Family Grows, by
Pamela L. Jordan, Scott M. Stanley, Howard J. Markman (Jossey-Bass,
2001). An excellent resource on how to prepare your marriage for baby.

*For Lesbian Parents: Your Guide to Helping Your Family Grow Up Happy, Healthy,
and Proud,* by Suzanne M. Johnson and Elizabeth O'Connor (Guilford
Press, 2001). Offers help on explaining lesbianism to children and
explores what lesbian parents can do to help children explain their
family situation to their peers.

Gay and Lesbian Parents' Coalition International, P.O. Box 50360, Washington, D.C. 20091. Phone 202-583-8029 for referrals to local support
groups, newsletters, and more. Visit http://www.milepost1.com/~gay-
dad/support.groups.html

How Men Have Babies, by Alan Thicke (Jodere Group, 2003). Comic relief for
fathers-to-be.

Pregnant Man: How Nature Makes Fathers Out of Men, by Gordon Churchwell
(Quill, 2001). A hilarious and scientific look at becoming a father.

Rookie Dad, by Rick Epstein (Hyperion, 1993). Diary of daddydom. Good
choice if your partner is afraid of infants.

The Expectant Father: Facts, Tips and Advice for Dads-to-Be, by Armin A. Brott
(Abbeville Press, 2001). An information-packed guide to all the emotional, financial, and physical changes dad-to-be may experience during
the course of his partner's pregnancy.

Websites:

Single Mothers by Choice
http://www.singlemothers.org

Nurture Mom
www.nurturemom.com

Parent's Place
http://www.ParentsPlace.com

Parenting Tool Box
www.parentingtoolbox.com

My Baby Connection
http://www.mybabyconnection.com/
ExpectingParents.html

It's Not All in Your Head

Surviving the Physical Discomfort of Pregnancy

When to Do It:

- When the idea of getting up to go to the bathroom one more time makes you ache with fatigue.

- When your ability to cope and occasionally chuckle has disappeared along with your ability to keep a meal down.

- If no one in your life believes you when you say, "I can't open my eyes. I'm really trying, but I can't."

- If you are positive you will never stop feeling this way.

What Is It?

If you are hugging the toilet, if you are furious at being as limp and mushy as two-week-old lettuce, if you are so constipated you feel like you are in labor, the most important things to remember, above all else, are:

> It isn't "in your head."

> It won't last forever.

> It doesn't mean you don't want your baby.

The idea that pregnancy-related discomfort, especially nausea and exhaustion, exist only in women's minds is the height of stupidity. When I had morning sickness, I felt guilty for being sick: "If I was a *real* woman, a *real* trooper, and *really* wanted my baby, I would feel great." You might feel a subtle competition to have a perfect

You'll Need:

Foods that appeal to you.

An occasional glimpse of acceptance and surrender.

A fluffy, feathery, fabulous sleeping, dreaming, napping, relaxing place. A nest of silken sheets, perfectly proportioned pillows, and freshly laundered comforters.

Permission to sleep the entire weekend away if you feel like it.

Black-out drapes if necessary.

Farting jokes.

pregnancy, because a perfect pregnancy implies you are a superior woman—not emotional or feeble—and truly want your baby. This too is absolute rubbish. *Your pregnancy is unique.* Everyone experiences some discomfort (along with some ambivalence and fear). Whether you have an "easy" pregnancy or a "difficult" one, it doesn't mean you are a bad mother, a less-than-competent woman, or anything else. Do not feel guilty! Do not let others make you feel guilty!

Unwanted criticism, lack of empathy, and guilt (self-imposed and imposed by others) commonly accompany morning sickness, severe exhaustion, and many of the other physical ailments you may experience. Your mate, relatives, and even friends might make you feel at fault, silly, or insane. To counter that, find someone who is sympathetic and has gone through this before you. I was very lucky to know Kristina, who was about six months ahead of me in the pregnancy experience and had suffered more severe discomfort. It was such a comfort to talk to her about how she felt and what had worked for her. The sicker you are, the more important empathetic support from other women becomes. Talking to women who have had difficult pregnancies is especially comforting if you must be hospitalized for vomiting or other complications.

See Appendix: Herbs, Oils, and Other Natural Comforters for more relief.

You don't have to suffer needlessly. You can be more comfortable if you are willing to take your discomfort seriously and give yourself time and attention. You deserve to take care of your basic needs. Keep repeating that to yourself when you feel overwhelmed with trying to take care of yourself.

What to Do:

Nausea

Nausea can be inconvenient, distressing, awkward, boring, nasty, and debilitating. One study found 50 to 80 percent of all pregnant women feel some degree of discomfort, while another study posited 36 to 76 percent of women feel sick all day long, especially in the first trimester. Very little is known about morning sickness, partly because medical research has barely begun to take it seriously (what a surprise). Some of you will not feel as if you are riding backward on a boat churning through twenty-five-foot waves with an outboard motor spewing exhaust into your face as you eat pickled herring and drink slightly soured milk. Great! Skip this section. For the rest, experiment. Morning sickness is so complex, and so little is known about it, that the solution that works for you will probably not work for your friend. Don't give up if something doesn't work. Try something else, try the same thing at a different time, try more or less of it, combine it with another remedy, try it again later, but *persist!* Second, *get help.* The combination of nausea and exhaustion can leave you so depleted you can't get to the store to buy sparkling water. Just reading this may exhaust you. *Get someone to run your errands.* Ask someone to cajole you into continuing to try different remedies. You will find some relief, maybe even a lot. And the hope of finding relief will keep you going until the queasiness is gone.

Extreme Vomiting

If you are suffering from extreme and constant vomiting, it is going to affect your attitude about your pregnancy and your ability to mother. This is completely normal. Do not suffer alone. *Tell your health care provider.* If he or she dismisses your suffering, go elsewhere. Trust me when I say you can feel better, you will not die, and getting support is critical. Do not get sucked into feeling like a failure or a whiner or a hypochondriac. Get help!

See Forming Your Support Team.

Practical Tips

The only antinausea formula that worked for me was to eat what I craved, no matter if it was junk food, hard to get, or expensive. Ask yourself, "What would make me feel better right now?" Miriam Erick, in her excellent book *No More Morning Sickness,* recommends going through the following list and asking yourself, "Would something salty make me feel better?" Or would something "sour, bitter, tart, sweet, crunchy/lumpy, soft/smooth, mushy, fruity, wet, dry, bland, spicy, aromatic, earthy, hot, cold, thin, or thick" make me feel better? The

See Food: Reinstating Instinct for additional help.

built-in mandate that women must care for everyone else can lead us not to get the food we need quickly enough to keep it down. One scenario: you crave a certain food. You've given yourself permission to eat whatever you want to get through this time (any calorie you can keep down is a nourishing calorie), but you need a turkey burger *now*. You don't want to ask anyone to get it for you, and your mate can't cook, so you try to prepare it, only to become too ill to eat from the odor or effort of cooking. *You've got to have someone help you.* The more severe your nausea, the more you must let go and ask for, arrange for, if possible pay for, and definitely demand help.

Become aware of what triggers your nausea. Smells of all kinds are the most common culprit. Tracey reported, "Three closed doors and several rooms stood between me and the refrigerator, but when Paul opened the door I could instantly smell if something had gone bad." Stress, driving, wearing glasses or contacts, bright lights, loud noises, crowds, reading, and hunger can all be triggers too. When you become ill, take in your surroundings. What time is it? What have you been doing, thinking, smelling, feeling in the last few minutes? Spend just a few seconds checking in with yourself. See if you can deduce what situations, substances, and smells to avoid. If you must encounter them, be ready with remedies. Trust your instincts. If you feel something is making you ill, get away from it as much as possible.

Specific remedies to experiment with:

- Eat bites of very hot or very cold foods—baked potato, shake, ice cream, or soup. Also try eating high protein snacks (or bites) every two hours.

- Sleep in a well-ventilated room, if possible with a window cracked.

- Make sure your kitchen is well ventilated so cooking odors don't penetrate the rest of your house. Cook with a window open.

- Don't be afraid to ask co-workers, family members, and your mate not to wear perfume, aftershave, hair treatments like mousse, or other smelly concoctions around you. You may have to unplug the office coffeepot, cover your nose with a handkerchief containing a few drops of lemon or lavender essential oil (or any smell you find comforting) when using the employee bathroom, or ask to have air fresheners removed. Approach these situations with tact, but don't suffer in silence.

- Kindly ask your mate to sleep in another room. Bodies give off odors during the night, and what your mate ate one day could make you ill the next morning.

- The smell of food on your hands might drive you mad. Try rubbing your hands with lemon. In fact, lemons in general are reported to help: suck a lemon, drink lemonade (a common craving), nibble lemon sorbet, or sniff a lemon.

- Avalon, mother of three and a potter, spent so much time in the bathroom, she made it her shrine. "I put pillows around the toilet for my knees, kept the bowl scrupulously clean so the smell wouldn't make me sicker, and even floated gardenias in the toilet water."

- Wear seasickness prevention bands, which can be purchased at a travel store, drugstore, or any place close to a marina. Designed for seasickness, they are positioned over acupressure points on your wrists. (They come with directions for placement.)

- Drink sparkling water with lime, caffeine-free cola, or ginger ale. Drink pineapple juice. Suck on ice cubes. Carry drinks with you in a small cooler. Carry cool, moist washcloths too; they are great comfort when you are stuck someplace getting sick.

- Carry double plastic grocery bags in your purse, car, and desk drawer to throw up in wherever you need to. Sue, mother of two and a saleswoman, suffered from severe nausea but had to maintain a busy travel schedule. Stuck at a sales conference at a round table in the middle of an enormous room listening to a long presentation, she survived by positioning plastic bags under the table and alerting a trusted co-worker sitting next to her to cover for her if she leaned under the table to throw up. "Tell anyone who asks I'm fixing my shoe." Sue also carried a toothbrush and toothpaste everywhere and immediately located the bathroom when entering a new environment.

IT'S NOT ALL
IN YOUR HEAD

*See Connecting with Your
Partner: Dependence and
Interdependence; and How
to Gracefully Ask for and
Accept Support.*

- Feeling ill for an extended period of time can put a strain on your relationship. One woman told me how she kept apologizing to her mate for waiting on her, which made both her and him feel worse. When it's offered, *accept the help*. This is your mate's baby too, and taking care of you is an important way for him or her to participate. Say thank you, but no apologies. Of course you are sorry you're sick, but *it is not your fault*. Draw your partner into a conversation about his or her feelings. Often, the overwhelming reality of becoming a parent, coupled with taking care of you (or suffering with you) and looking after the daily business of life, can be almost too much to handle. Talk about dependency issues. Talk about how you will divide the work in preparation for your baby. Talk about your hopes and fears.

- See a medical professional about B_{12} injections with extra C. Acupuncture from a trained professional who treats pregnant women can help with many pregnancy ailments. And finally, there's hospitalization. As one woman told me, "I wish I hadn't resisted going in for so long. Getting that IV for forty-eight hours helped *a lot*. But I thought if I went in earlier, I would be a failure." Once again, a reluctance to ask for and accept help can be a real hindrance to relief.

Exhaustion

You will probably experience bouts of exhaustion throughout your pregnancy, with the worst being in the first three months. This is because you are creating the placenta, which will take over much of the baby-making work for you later in the pregnancy so you will not feel like Wily Coyote flattened by the Roadrunner for the millionth time.

Don't Fight the Fatigue

If you spend your energy maintaining you feel great, or if you spend your energy worrying about why you are so tired, you will become even more spent. This too shall pass. In the meantime, nap. Give yourself permission to go to bed, no matter what time of the day or evening. If you are beating yourself up—"I should have more energy. There is so much to do at work"—stop! I promise, you will feel better, but it will happen in a much more enjoyable and faster way if you stop wasting precious time worrying. Make sleep a priority.

That means sleep is more important than doing the laundry or even taking your other child(ren) to the park. If you have a toddler, tell him or her, "You have to nap because mommy has to nap. This won't last forever. I still love you, but I'll be a lot nicer if I rest." (It's worth a try.) Get a baby-sitter so you can doze. If life is too crazy at home, check into a cheap motel and sleep for twelve hours (make sure you get a quiet room).

If you drive to work, nap in your car during your lunch hour or break. You can bring a travel alarm or digital watch to wake you up. Or if you have an office and can close your door, bring an exercise mat and light blanket and stretch out on the floor during your lunch hour. Employee lounges can be restful if you bring a Walkman or head-phones to block out noise. A sleeping mask or soft bag filled with herbs to block out light is also handy. (Yes, your fellow employees may scoff. Flip them the universal sign of scorn and keep on napping.)

Use your exhaustion to help you set limits with others.

Have your iron level checked. Low iron levels are very common, and iron supplements can help relieve the sensation of crawling through Vaseline.

See Nurturing Yourself During Pregnancy: Cut to the Chase.

Exercise

If you are healthy, forcing yourself to exercise, even for ten minutes, honestly does help fatigue. Prenatal exercise classes can be worth every penny, and many women I interviewed told me their prenatal exercise class was the best thing they did for themselves. The exercises you do can help relieve exhaustion and even nausea, but also being around other yawning, farting, dragging-their-butts women can make you feel less alone (as long as the windows are open).

IT'S NOT ALL
IN YOUR HEAD

See I Am a Body Without a
Brain: Practical Advice for
more exhaustion ideas.

Try this simple yoga pose: Fold a blanket once. Put the blanket against a wall, put your hips on it, with your butt against the wall, and straighten your legs, letting them rest along the wall, feet relaxed. Roll your shoulder blades under you, opening your chest. Breathe deeply for five minutes. (This can also help with gas and constipation.)

Getting Comfortable in Bed

Nothing really makes you as comfortable as you would be if you weren't trying to sleep with a writhing hip-hop dancer in your womb, but try these techniques anyway:

Surround yourself with *lots* of pillows. One extra-thin pillow for the first six months tucked between your legs or under your belly can feel great. Those great big body pillows can be helpful in the last months, but try one out in the store because it might be too bulky for you. (Also, it does take up a lot of room and tends to get between you and your bed partner.) One woman swore by those tiny little airline pillows for tucking into "all those little spaces near the end that need support."

If indigestion or breathlessness is waking you or keeping you up, try sleeping propped up, with pillows surrounding you on all sides and under your knees.

If you have pain in your hips, thighs, or lower back, place thin pillows under your hips, take extra calcium, and get a massage from someone who is familiar with pregnancy.

If you want to sleep on your stomach later in pregnancy, put several pillows under your hips and one or two under your head and chest, so you make a cave for your tummy.

See Nurturing Yourself
During Pregnancy: Zen
and the Art of Peeing; and
Postbirth Nourishment:
Surviving and Thriving for
help with broken sleep
after the baby arrives.

Accept changing sleep patterns and frequent trips to the bathroom as what they are: preparation for feeding babykins in the middle of the night and compulsively listening for your baby's breathing. I hated waking up early in the morning, but I managed to pause on daybreak bathroom ventures to appreciate the sunrise and, as sentimental as this sounds, to watch my husband sleep.

Constipation and Gas

Gas and constipation are both caused by a slowdown in your digestive system because your musculature is relaxing. The same hormones that are going to make it possible for your bones and muscles to relax sufficiently to let your baby out are already working, and that can make your bowels sluggish, which leads to constipation, which leads to gas. Gas can also be worsened by your change in diet. You may be eating better than you ever have before, but as many vegetarians will tell you, all those lovely broccoli florets and protein-packing bowls of beans and rice can pack a wallop.

A bad case of gas or constipation can be very painful and can even feel like labor. Some women worry that the pressure will hurt the baby. It won't. What will help is to *relax*. Again, don't waste energy fighting the discomfort. An especially nasty bout of constipation can actually be good practice for labor, because the pain comes in waves. Breathe. Tell yourself you will pass this brick. Listen to a relaxation tape, have someone baby you, and drink plenty of fluids. If you are at all worried, call your health care provider.

Eating quickly, gulping your food, or eating with tense, uptight companions can increase your gas because you are swallowing too much air. You will soon be obsessed with swallowing air—how much air your baby swallows affects the amount of burping, spitting up, and gas you have to contend with—so practice on yourself now.

Practical tips:

Start the day with a glass of warm water.

Visiting a chiropractor can be useful for relieving a blocked or sluggish bowel.

Yoga can be helpful, as can going for a short walk or any gentle form of exercise. You can do these two poses until you feel too ungainly and unsteady:

The Half Shoulder Stand is good for constipation. Lie on your back with your legs straight. Inhale as you raise your legs, your feet pointing up. Exhale as you continue the upward motion by bringing your hips up, bending your knees if necessary, while placing your hands under your hips to support yourself. Your feet will be pointing over your head. Breathe and maintain this position for as long as it feels good. To release, bend your knees, and slowly lower your feet and hips to the ground.

Try the Shoulder Stand for gas relief. Lie on your back, with your shoulders on a blanket that has been folded twice. Your head and neck relax off the blanket onto the floor. Inhaling, raise your legs, bending your knees if that feels better. Exhale as you lift your hips off the floor. Support your hips with your hands, resting your weight on your elbows. Exhale, lifting your legs as high as is comfortable for you, never straining. Hold this position as long as feels comfortable. Very gradually reverse direction.

Small, frequent meals cut down on gas, fatigue, and mood swings. You may feel like you are eating all the time (you are), and you will get annoyed, but it helps.

Talk to your health care provider about taking a break from your pre-natal vitamins and any other supplements for three days. Not all vitamins are created equal, and they can often be the culprit in both excessive gas and constipation. If they are, seek out a nutritionist who can recommend a more digestible supplement. Or visit several health foods stores and ask an informed person what he or she recommends. Or look up vitamins in your library magazine database.

Avoid gas-causing foods for a few days before a big event, riding on a airplane, attending a movie, or putting yourself in any other enclosed space. Broccoli, beans, kale—many of the things you are supposed to eat—can make you "snap, crackle, pop." Carbonated drinks, fermented foods like cheese and soy sauce, and milk if you are lactose intolerant may also be contributing to your gas.

If All Else Fails, Laugh

Wear a T-shirt that says "Don't tailgate" or "Warning: Flammable." In exercise class, stay in the back of the room. Practice sidling up to open windows without being detected. Stay away from very quiet environments. Learn some good farting jokes.

Resources:

The Morning Sickness Companion, by Elizabeth Kaledin, (Griffin, 2003). A humorous and very helpful manual to softening the effects.

The Natural Pregnancy Book: Herbs, Nutrition and Other Holistic Choices, by Aviva Jill Romm (Celestial Arts, 2003). Like having your own personal herbalist and midwife at your side. Follows your journey from conception to birth, describing herbs that can promote and maintain a healthy pregnancy and the basics of a healthy diet.

The Pregnancy Bed Rest Book: A Survival Guide for Expectant Mothers and Their Families, by Amy E. Tracy (Berkley Pub Group, 2001). Ideas on how to survive during bedrest without going crazy or blaming yourself.

When Pregnancy Isn't Perfect, by Laurie Rich (Larata Press, 1996). *Hyperemesis gravidarum* is the medical term for what 1 to 3 in 1,000 pregnant women suffer from. Also offers help for bed rest, C-section recovery, and other pregnancy complications.

Websites:

Morning Sickness
http://www.sosmorningsickness.com

Muti Oil Morning Sickness Relief Stick
www.Mutioils.Com

Preggie Pops
www.Preggiepop.Com

Food

You'll Need:

A straightforward book on nutrition (See Resources.)

A food diary for several weeks.

Foods you crave.

When to Do It:

- If you are feeling anxious or confused about nutrition.

- When you feel that you are gaining too much weight too fast, or too little weight too slowly.

- If food has been a painful or touchy issue for you in the past.

- If you've always imagined pregnancy as a deliciously relaxed time in which you could eat whatever you wish.

What Is It?

When I found out I was pregnant, my first thought was, "This is impossible. I can't be a parent, I'm not ready. I'm not grown up." My second thought was, "This means I can *eat*. This means I can eat *a lot* of *anything* I want—after all, ice cream is full of calcium!"

Oh, how naive I was! I had no idea how overwhelming the question of food becomes when you are pregnant. Eating right, eating enough, eating too much, not wanting to eat, a smorgasbord of guilt, a deluge of advice, and so many conflicting opinions over what is actually good nutrition. Nor did I realize how directly I was going to come into conflict with how food comforts me. After I read one popular book on pregnancy, I felt like I would be eating twenty-three hours a day but nothing I particularly liked. No sugar said another book, no chocolate said my first midwife, two eggs and a quart of milk said another book. I was being sentenced to ten months of hospital food. Overcome with a sense of "I'll never be able to do this right, this is too much!" I headed promptly to the bakery for several large chocolate chip cookies.

Sheila Kitzinger, author of many childbirth books, puts it well in *Your Baby, Your Way:*

I believe that there are several things wrong with the way in which a good deal of counseling about diet in pregnancy is offered: it is often very dogmatic—implying that you must drink two pints of milk a day and have liver three times a week or you are starving your baby. It is also often presented as exclusively of benefit to the unborn baby, *not the mother.* She is supposed to ignore her own preferences and put the right raw materials in so that she will turn out a quality controlled product at the end of nine months. It is as if she were a machine to make a baby. If for any reason she does not stick to the rules, she feels guilty. [Italics mine.]

Almost all the women I interviewed had plenty to say about eating during pregnancy. Either they were very strict about how they were eating, or they were as confused as I was. Giving our unborn children good nutrition is vital, and attitudes today are far better than they were in the late sixties, when women were still given diuretics and low-calorie diets and told to gain only twenty-four pounds no matter what their body type, but intense pressure concerning food is still common. You may find yourself feeling anything from:

Slightly guilty ("I had pizza for dinner. Is that high in protein? I shouldn't have had it. Too much fat. I should have had brown rice and broccoli instead.")

to

Very uptight ("I had 39 grams of protein for lunch and 19 for breakfast. Well, I'm not actually sure about breakfast because the bakery didn't know the exact count on the bran muffin, even after I asked to speak to the baker, but I can guess, just this once. That leaves 22 for dinner—that should be easy. Now, what about my calcium count?")

to

Full-on rebellion ("This is the one time in my life when it is okay to eat, and I'm going to enjoy every minute of it. Who cares how much weight I gain? I'll lose it when I breast-feed.")

None of these reactions is very comforting. Nor are any of them likely to lead to an enhanced sense of self-esteem, self-celebration, or a healthier relationship with food.

There is another way. At perhaps no other time in your life will your body so clearly tell you what it needs. The way to find peace with food, during pregnancy and beyond, is by reinstating your instincts. Pregnancy turns your instincts on full alert. The trick is to quiet down and tune in to them, while using solid information as a comparison point.

What to Do:

Reinstating Instinct

A doctor said to a pregnant friend, "I wish all women could think about food like a pregnant woman." What the doctor meant was a pregnant body speaks up *very* loudly, telling you what it needs. Reinstating your instinct means you listen to the inherent, intuitive body wisdom, the inner voice that will tell you what your body and your baby need.

Listening to your inner voice of bodily wisdom can be difficult. You may not feel like eating (first and last trimester). You don't have time. Food is so wonderful to turn to in times of distress (and pregnancy can hand you plenty of distress), making it hard to know the difference between a habitual craving and your body telling you what it honestly needs. When you do stop to listen, you may not hear anything because your instincts may have been damaged by years of over-controlling what you eat or feeling guilty about how much you eat or what you weigh. Or perhaps you are just overwhelmed and confused about eating during pregnancy—does it have to be such a complicated endeavor? The ideas below can help you focus on your intuitive body wisdom.

Sit down someplace quiet when you are just beginning to be hungry. Do not wait until full hunger sets in, because hunger leaves you with no patience and tends to trigger the inner voice of habit, not instinct.

Take thirty seconds to breathe deeply and focus on how your body feels. Are you tense anywhere? Are you tired? Do you have any awareness of what your baby is doing? Take a few moments to increase your bodily awareness. Then, ask yourself, "What does my baby need to eat right now?" See what menu ideas float into your head. Whatever occurs to you, act on it. Encourage your inner wisdom by taking it seriously. But what if something occurs to you that isn't supposed to be good for the baby, like a double espresso with a shot of whiskey? Then take ten seconds more to ask yourself, "What have I been denying myself that I really need?" This second question allows you to make the connection with your own needs and how they are tied to food as comfort. Often, the answer won't be food as much as something else— say rest or thinking about yourself for a while instead of your children or your partner or your job. Again, don't dismiss what comes into your mind, even if the idea seems very fragile and dim. This method will not work if you say, "Well of course I need more rest. But who has time? I have to get this project done before the baby comes." It is this core denial of our needs that sets us up to be the kind of mothers we don't want to be: selfless, bitter, controlling martyrs. It is also the kind of attitude that leads to burnout, pregnancy complications such as preterm labor, and a general lack of a good time. (I don't mean to sound stern. I just know how insidious that voice can be, pushing us when we need to slow down and be good to ourselves. I want to give you a voice that is just as strong to counteract it.)

If you don't feel like concentrating on the baby's needs, ask yourself instead, "What does my body need to eat right now?" This is a different, but equally valuable, question. Experiment with both questions and see which works best for you.

Encourage your senses. Take a walk through a farmer's market and sample different kinds of strawberries, oranges, or apples. See if you can taste the differences between varieties. Touch different foods and feel the textures. Take in the colors and scents. Listen to the dialogue in your head, without judgment. What are you telling yourself about the healthy foods you see? Or visit a large health food store and spend some time browsing, taking in all the different possibilities. (This is obviously not a good exercise to do if smells are making you ill. Save this for when you are feeling better.)

Strike the word *cheat* from your vocabulary. If too many foods are off-limits to you, eventually (and probably regularly) you will find yourself eating them, usually in larger quantities than you would wish. It is simply a law of the universe: what is forbidden becomes irresistible, the focus of your energy and thoughts. Also, the word *cheat* conjures up feelings of being a bad girl, of being on a diet, all of which are disempowering. What you want to create during your pregnancy is a feeling of empowerment and self-love. A cheat doesn't sound like someone who loves herself.

A Backup Plan

It can feel risky to trust your instincts. It helps to have a backup plan—some simple guidelines to check yourself against. It also helps to discover what some of your comfort foods are and to build these foods into your diet.

Keep a diet diary for one week, during which you try to follow your inner wisdom but also live your normal life. You eat what your mother-in-law made for Sunday dinner, you get too hungry and go crazy at the deli, you come home to find there is nothing but peanut butter and jelly for dinner. Be scrupulous; write down *everything*. This isn't about feeling guilty. It's about finding out you are doing a better job than you think.

After the week is over, study your diary. First, how do you think you are doing? Trust yourself: what do you think you need more or less of? How true have you been to your own inner needs instead of giving in to stress or the needs of others, for example, eating what your family wants? There is no need for blame. Just become mindful of your eating habits. Jot down any notes you can think of about changes you would like to make in your diet. Again, trust yourself. Next, tally up the nutritional value of what you ate using a nutritional counter (like *The Quick and Easy Counter for Pregnancy*). Add up the whole week instead of each day; it is less stressful and more accurate to go by the week, since one day you do well, the next a little less. Add up how much protein you ate, how much calcium, how many fresh veggies and fruit. Don't worry about precision. You may find yourself lacking in one or two areas. That's normal. Make a note of what foods you want to add or delete from your diet, then post notes around your kitchen and office containing food suggestions. Then let it rest. Your body will do the rest.

If you are still feeling in doubt, consult with your health care provider. The reason I put this last is if you rely too much on your doctor or midwife, you may feel like a little girl who has been told what to do. In addition, some doctors still impose unnecessarily strict weight gain limits for low-risk pregnancies, as well as employing guilt to keep you in line ("You keeping eating like this and you'll never lose the weight"). As long as you are primarily eating a balanced, nutritious diet and keeping the Ho-Hos to a minimum, the amount of weight you gain is perfect. Truly listen to your body, with a few slips now and then, and compare this to some basic nutritional guidelines, and all will be well.

What are your comfort foods—the foods you crave so loudly that when you are tired or hungry or stressed, what you hear is "I need a vanilla milk shake" no matter what your body really needs? For me, comfort is chocolate, even more enticing because it is forbidden. For you, it might be cookies-and-cream ice cream, hazelnut coffee, or McDonald's french fries. It is true these aren't the best things for you or your baby, but are you going to feel deprived if you rule them out completely? Will you then go off the deep end and eat or drink too much and then feel very guilty, which will trigger another binge later? Make an honest, specific deal with yourself. For example: I will have chocolate only once a week in an amount I feel is safe. Or, I will eat ice cream every third day. Create a realistic plan you can stick to. Strike a balance between discipline and desire.

Note: Caffeine and alcohol are not good for the baby. It is up to you to learn and decide what the risk to the fetus is versus what you need. This weighing of your needs versus the baby's will go on your entire life, or at least for the next eighteen years. The key is "Do you really *need* this?" Sometimes the answer will be "Yes, I need this food to maintain my sanity." Other times it will be "No, I sure want it, but I don't need it." It is this kind of discernment you are after. (If you think you have an addiction that precludes your making an informed choice, seek help *immediately*.)

Best Nutrition Trick

This easy nutrition trick is from labor support and home birth advocate Laura Whitney. This is a good way to double-check your eating habits. Or if all this talk about "body wisdom" makes you feel like belting out Carole King's "I Feel like a Natural Woman" and braiding your leg hairs, this approach may appeal to you more.

LAURA'S PREGNANCY DIET COLOR WHEEL "When I was pregnant, I made preparing meals an aesthetic experience . . . an artistic challenge! For at least one meal each day (usually dinner, sometimes lunch and dinner) I would challenge myself to prepare a plate with at least five colors on it." This is more than aesthetics; this means you're getting the range of vitamins and minerals you need.

Red/Purple

Tomato, red bell pepper, rhubarb, beets, red cabbage, strawberries, cherries, plums, aduki beans, kidney beans, new potatoes, eggplant

Yellow/Orange

Yellow bell pepper, spaghetti squash, butternut/acorn squash, carrots, millet, corn, cornmeal, eggs, red lentils, melon, banana, peaches, orange, papaya, apricots

White

Cauliflower, mushrooms, potato, pasta, rice, white beans, tofu, jicama, whole grain bread, onions, garlic, turnips, fish, chicken, cottage cheese, yogurt, cheese

Broccoli, string beans, peas, lima beans, zucchini, artichoke, asparagus, lettuce, cabbage, spinach, beet greens, kale, Swiss chard, celery, bean sprouts, cucumber, green pepper

Brown

Brown rice, bulgur wheat, whole wheat anything, nuts, seeds, wheat germ, lentils, pinto beans, black beans, meat, crackers, miso, oats, raisins, figs, prunes

This method works when you are "grazing," eating small meals every few hours, too. Just keep a running tally of colors, and toward the end of the day eat any colors you haven't consumed yet.

I Would Like to Change My Eating Habits

For those of us who have a conflicted relationship with food, approaching nutrition during pregnancy as a time to heal can be liberating. It can also be necessary if we are to head off behavior that may make it difficult to eat in a healthy way. However, if you are feeling overwhelmed or stressed about food, disregard this section.

Sit down with your journal or paper and a pen. Write for five minutes on the question "What would I change about my eating habits if I could?" Push past your first reactions and obvious answers by keeping your hand moving, even if you are writing nonsense.

Study what you wrote. What one area are you willing to take on during this transformational time? Write down one idea for change. Under it, write all the reasons why you haven't changed in the past. Then, write all the reasons why pregnancy is the best time to try, and then why pregnancy is the worst time to change. Finally, decide on three small, specific actions you are willing to take to instigate this change, to make it real, and write these on your calendar, only one for each of the next three weeks. This is one woman's response:

I would like to eat fewer processed foods.

I haven't changed in the past because I'm too busy, I like junk food, it makes me feel good, it reminds me of my childhood, I get too hungry and I can't think of what else I want, it is always available, my partner buys it, it's too expensive to eat health food, I don't believe I deserve organic foods, sugar really isn't that bad for you.

Pregnancy is a good time to try to change because my body has such clear cravings, the books say processed foods are the worst, chemicals in those foods could be bad for the baby even if they aren't for me, these foods could make me fatter, I want to change, fresh fruit actually sounds good to me.

Pregnancy is a bad time to try to change because I'm nauseated, I'm tired and don't want to think, we are trying to save money and I don't want to spend more for food now, my husband is doing more of the shopping and it is too much of a struggle to tell him what to buy, I get so hungry I'll eat anything, I feel very close to my childhood and I want familiar foods, I crave sugar, I feel like being bad not good sometimes.

Three specific, small actions I am willing to take over the next three weeks are keep a food diary for one week without trying to change my eating habits, limiting myself to one Coke per week; going shopping at the health food store with coupons.

Avoid big changes; they will cause too much anxiety. Also, know that it may not be possible to stick to your plan. That's okay. It is the slow process of becoming aware of your beliefs and habits and making tiny changes that brings you to eat in a way that is more self-nurturing for you and your unborn child. That's all you need to do. It is more than enough.

Survival Tips

In the beginning, when you need to eat, you need to eat *now*. Near the end, it is often much more comfortable to eat many small meals. But trying to eat that way and live your life can be cumbersome. I would get ready to leave the house and think, "But I haven't eaten in two hours. #@%&#, got to stop and eat first." Carrying snacks is one answer. Buy or devise several different-sized reusable snack and fluid carriers to make it easy to pack food and drink. Have more than one of each size so that if you are too exhausted at night to wash one out, you have a clean container to pack in the morning. (Being constantly prepared with snacks is another subtle way pregnancy prepares you for motherhood.) Scatter snacks throughout your life: at work, in the car, in your purse, in the diaper bag if you already have a child, in your backpack. What to take for snacks? Whole wheat pretzels, carrots, broccoli pieces, red bell pepper slices, trail mix, dried (nonsulfite) fruit, crackers and hard cheese, grapes, oranges, high-protein bars (try a health food store), yogurt-covered nuts, and fig bars all have good nutritional value and keep for a few days. (Hiding food does have its down side. I found a plastic baggie with black and green slime under my car seat months after Lillian was born.)

When you are feeling energetic, research the healthiest take-out options in your neighborhood. Collect menus and figure out which meal choices have the most vegetables, the most protein, the least amount of added fat, and that appeal to your most common cravings. You may need to call the restaurant during off-hours to find out how they prepare a certain dish to ascertain fat or additives you don't want. Highlight your choices and put them in a folder near the phone for emergency help on nights when you are exhausted and about to gasp your last from lack of food. (Keep these menus for your postpartum convenience.)

Buy bottles, decanters, or water pitchers and place them on your desk, your bedside table, and your favorite lounging spot. It makes it easier to drink enough water and you'll really appreciate them if you breastfeed.

Get help. Everyone talks about needing people to come in and cook after the baby is born, but pregnant women often need almost as much help in the beginning, especially if you have other children or if you are confined to bed with complications.

See How to Gracefully Ask for and Accept Support; and Forming Your Support Team.

If your work schedule, other children, or exhaustion makes it too difficult to eat in a way that nourishes you, consider whether you can afford:

- Washed, prepared salad mix or cut-up raw veggies

- Frozen entrees from the health food store

- Premixed healthy salads or entrees from the supermarket or health store deli (ask what the ingredients are—watch out for extra fat and additives)

- Lunch meats sans sodium nitrates

- Prepared juice shakes

- Cans of health food store beans mixed with rice, which you can make in a large pot and keep in the refrigerator

- Someone to come in to cook once a week, making a casserole, a big pot of soup, brown rice, and perhaps cutting up and bagging all sorts of vegetables for easy steaming, salads, and snacking. It may sound way too expensive, but do some investigating before ruling it out. During this food-intensive time, you might consider giving something else up temporarily (I don't mean car insurance but maybe yard help, car wash, or dry cleaning) to have the money to pay for help in the kitchen.

Resources:

Eating Expectantly: A Practical and Tasty Guide to Prenatal Nutrition, by Bridget Swinney and Tracey Anderson (Meadowbrook, 2000). Good choice if you don't like to cook, not as good if you are a vegan or vegetarian.

Eating for Pregnancy: An Essential Guide to Nutrition with Recipes for the Whole Family, by Catherine Jones and Rose Ann Hudson (Marlowe and Company, 2003). Balances optimum and unnecessary weight gain concerns, outlines how to get enough protein, how to eat if you are diabetic, vegetarian or vegan, and provides over a 100 recipes.

Every Woman's Guide to Eating During Pregnancy, by Martha Rose Shulman and Jane Davis, M.D. (Houghton Mifflin, 2002). Written by an award winning cookbook author and a doctor. Excellent recipes – a good choice for women who like to cook.

The Mother of All Pregnancy Books: The Ultimate Guide to Conception, Birth, and Everything In-Between, by Ann Douglas (John Wiley and Sons, 2002). A mom-friendly guide to conception, pregnancy, birth, and beyond. Nutritional guidance too.

Comforting Clothing
and Other Sensual Strategies

When to Do It:

- When Monday morning or Saturday night finds you panicking and saying, "I just fit into these pants two days ago!"

- If you have a limited budget (who doesn't?).

- If dressing well is an important part of your job.

- When you want to glory in your luminescent splendor.

What Is It?

It can become quite an aggravating issue: What to wear. How to feel attractive. How to keep everyone at work from focusing on your belly. How to go to a party with all your nonpregnant friends without feeling jealous and whalelike. "Fashion," "beauty," and "How do I look?" can loom large in your life as they haven't since adolescence. And maternity clothes are expensive! So here are a few tricks to keep you feeling as beautiful as you already are and as comfortable as possible.

What to Do:

Making Do in the Beginning

The beginning. The time of thickening, when you consider wearing a T-shirt that says, "I'm not fat, I'm pregnant." Also a time of plunging cleavage, which is cause for celebration for some ("I've got boobs!"),

You'll Need:

A plan.

Friends to borrow from.

Large, fun, funky, wild accessories.

Very good, very supportive bras.

Discount, thrift, and maternity stores.

mourning for others ("How could they get any bigger?"). The time of
dark circles under the eyes and a severely churning stomach. We won't
call it the first trimester, because for some of us it lasts through the
second or longer. Everyone gains weight and "shows" differently.
Here are some coping ideas for your beginning, however long that
might last.

It can be depressing and time consuming to constantly shuffle through
your favorite clothes that you can no longer fit into. One of the few
boons of maternity dressing is simplicity. Get a large cardboard box.
Line it with scented tissue paper. Go through your closet and move to
the front everything that has an elastic waist, every big blouse, sweater,
pullover, empire waist, or coat dress, anything you can wear for the
next few months. Pack away the clothes that are already too small.
Postnatal and after you've lost most of the weight (yes, it will happen!), you can unpack your clothes and it will (almost) be like going
on a shopping spree. Store the boxes in the back of your closet, under
your bed, or in the attic or garage. Good suits and dresses can be hung
in the coat closet or your mate's closet if you don't want to fold them.

I didn't realize how long I could wear "regular" clothes—elastic-waist
skirts and pants, big tops, and even fitted blouses under overalls. I
didn't realize I could shop in regular stores and that certain clothes
would fit until almost the end. I also didn't realize I wouldn't be able
to button my jeans by the end of the first month. Tip number one:
get creative with what you have. Wait to go shopping for maternity
clothes as long as you can. It is common in the beginning of your
pregnancy to buy more than you need, to buy things you hate two
days later, or to buy circus tents. However, it can be useful to shop for
accessories, underwear, and big T-shirts early on. I bought inexpensive
cotton bikini briefs one size larger and wore those below my belly
(they got so below, they almost disappeared), throwing them out afterward. Some women prefer over-the-belly maternity panties. Buy one
pair and experiment. Several kinds of underwear styles are available,
so if neither bikinis nor "balloon" pants feel good, try a maternity
store. Big T-shirts bought at the discount store are versatile throughout
your pregnancy.

About accessories: almost every pregnancy book discusses them. I thought it was silly. Until I too became obsessed with scarves—anything to relieve the boredom of my same three outfits. Tip two: the bigger the accessory, the better. Why? Proportion.

Tip three: no matter how many times your mother drummed into your head "Never a borrower or lender be," borrow *everything* you can, including accessories that aren't your usual style. However, do be careful whom you borrow from. If you have a friend who bought an incredible maternity wardrobe and will freak out if one or two things come back worn or stained, borrow things you will wear only once or twice. You need someone like Tracey, who said, "If you won't use it comfortably, don't take it. If I get it back, great. If I don't, so what." You might want to keep a list of what you borrow from whom because you may forget. Offer some of your regular clothes in exchange. Borrowing is especially important in cold weather when buying a new coat for the last two months would be very expensive. Raid your dad's or partner's closet!

For skirts and pants with waists, buy a few heavy-duty rubber bands. Hook the rubber band through the buttonhole and secure the other end around the button. Undo any zippers until you are comfortable. It does feel precarious at first but works pretty well. Carry extra rubber bands with you!

Buying Clothes: What Works Best

Planning carefully is your best strategy in making dollars stretch and staving off the uglies. Pretend you are going on a ten-month trip and you can take only one suitcase. The rules: Everything needs to be easy to care for, because of exhaustion and because maternity clothes are washed four to five times more often than a regular garment (so beware of dry-clean-only tags because it can get expensive). Separates in two or three complementary colors work best. Have two pairs of comfortable shoes that go with everything (this is less important if your feet don't swell because of course your old shoes will still fit). Plus add a few accessories to break the tedium. Best-case scenario: invite over a

See Forming Your Support Team on meeting women who have maternity clothes.

friend who has been pregnant recently to help. Lay out what you already own—big T-shirts, jogging pants, shoes, scarves. Consider:

- What kind of situation *must* I look good for?

- What styles and fabrics would make me most comfortable and feel most beautiful?

- Are there any special events coming up? (*Do not* wait until right before a black-tie event or wedding to plan what to wear.)

You probably can't afford to buy clothes for every situation in which you wish to look ravishing, so concentrate on where you must look your best: work, public speaking, when you pick your old friend up at the airport, business trips.

Remember, everything has to fit in one suitcase; keep it simple. You might be surprised how just one or two hours spent planning will make this whole clothing hassle less stressful and depressing.

Bras

It is imperative to buy several excellent bras as soon as possible. Don't wait and don't skimp; buy two of the best bras you can afford. Kristina wanted someone to "treat me like a mother," so she visited a posh department store's lingerie department and found a knowledgeable clerk to measure her for a proper fit. What kind of bra to buy? One that covers your entire breast, supports you enough so you barely jiggle when walking fast, and has well-padded straps. Some women swear by maternity bras, which I loved and which offer four sets of hooks and longer straps for greater adjustability. Other women buy regular underwire bras with bigger cups and more support. Do not push yourself into skimpy or undersized bras; you will be uncomfortable and this can cause extra stress to your breast tissue.

For a nursing bra, wait until close to your due date to invest. Buy a bra one to two cup sizes larger than you are right now, but the same chest size (like 36). Buy only one or two bras now because you can't be sure what size your breasts will settle at or what type of bra will feel most comfortable.

Waist Down

Maternity shops are best for bottoms—skirts, shorts, and pants. Buy in
your prepregnancy size, and these garments are supposed to fit until
the end (it usually works—except sometimes at the very end). What
you do in the meantime is roll the waistband over. If you buy bottoms
at large-size stores, you might find the stomach and butt fit, but your
thighs are lost. Investigate these stores but beware of the overall fit.
Inspect your usual clothing stores for elastic-waist pants, skirts, and
shorts that are too long from crotch to waist. You roll the waistband
down when you're small, then up as your belly expands.

Check out thrift and discount stores. Several large discount chains
offer excellent, inexpensive maternity basics, like leggings and cotton
pullovers. Visit the men's department too; drawstring athletic shorts
for working out, T-shirts, and boxer shorts come in handy (and you
can give them to your mate when you're done). Thrift stores take
patience, creativity, and repeat visits. Consignment stores have become
popular and can offer great bargains. Beware: because you are getting a
good bargain, it is easy to go a little crazy and buy things you don't
really need or like.

Putting It All Together

Slimmer bottoms with big tops work better than miles of flowing fabric, unless you are tall. The best maternity piece I found was a slip top
sewn to a straight black skirt. The slip has adjustable Velcro straps so
nothing tightens around your waist and the hemline doesn't ride up as
you get rounder. If you sew, you can make one by sewing a man's tank
top (size large) to a piece of fabric wide enough to wrap loosely
around your hips. The tank top should hang loosely to your hips,
where the fabric begins. Stretch the tank to match the width of the
skirt fabric when sewing. Top with anything from oversized sweaters
to your partner's flannel shirts.

If how you dress at work is of stellar importance and/or you are worried about your job security because of your pregnancy, you are going
to have to consider investing more than usual in clothing—both in

dollars and in time. If money is not an issue, do all your shopping in a good maternity shop or by catalog. Tricks to get by with only two maternity suits: for variety, wear regular blouses, worn unbuttoned from the waist down under a vest or sweater; T-shirts with a large, silk scarf tied biblike around your neck and pinned to your T-shirt at the waist (drawback: you have to keep your jacket on); a scarf pinned to one shoulder and tied on the opposite hip, over a jacket or blouse; sweeping your hair up or back or any way that is different so instead of everyone noticing the suit, they notice your hair. Other working women told me taking great care of their hands and buying new makeup helped them feel more elegant.

Weirdest idea: wear lounging clothes or glorified pajamas out of the house. Can be especially effective for a dress-up event. Very comfortable.

Full-length leotards in bright colors under large sweaters feel great because the leotard hugs your uterus, giving it support, but doesn't bind. Loose, flowing dresses that you adjust with a clip work well. The best dresses have empire waists or no waists and buttons to just below your breasts. Then you can wear the dress when you nurse but you don't have to worry about buttons popping open over your belly.

Comfort ideas from women I interviewed:

- Cowboy boots with everything for a tall, slim feeling.

- Leggings and big sweaters as a uniform.

- Natural fibers only—nothing with polyester in it.

- Hire a seamstress. Take several old skirts or pants and have expandable panels sewn in the top.

- No hose!

- Only loose dresses with no waistbands, even during exercise.

- More frequent haircuts and wild hair accessories.

- Regular facials to help with skin changes.

Labor Clothes

You will want your most comforting, soothing, and reassuring clothing
on or around you when you are in labor. Nancy bought a lacy white
nightgown. Stacey bought huge cotton T-shirts and heavy socks. She
wanted to be able to change after showers and when she became
sweaty. Margot preferred her oldest flannel nightgown and robe, which
she discarded for nakedness halfway through. Rhonda wore two hospital gowns, one on backward to close the gap, and got a prelabor
pedicure. "I studied my perfectly manicured toes during contractions.
It distracted me." Another woman bought a soft, cotton shawl to drape
around her.

Consider briefly what would make you feel powerful, unrestricted,
and beautiful. When you watch birthing videos in childbirth class,
make a note of what the women are wearing, if anything. Think about
your modesty level—what will allow you to labor effectively and still
feel comfortable?

After labor, especially if you end up in a hospital for several days
(but this is also nice at home), it can be especially comforting to have
something beautiful to slip into. If you will be nursing, keep in mind
easy breast availability. Your favorite sweats and a new nursing T-shirt
might make you feel less like an invalid. Consider putting together a
little bag of luxurious toiletries for the hospital—samples of shampoo,
conditioner, a tiny special soap, and scented lotion. (If you are having
a home or birthing-center birth, have these special treats laid out in
your bathroom.)

Postpartum

What will you wear after the baby? This can be a real dilemma because
you have no idea what your size will be. How big will you be right
after labor? What about at two weeks? Three months? If or when you
go back to work? The best bet is to pull out clothes from your early
pregnancy, the things you wore a lot the first few months but haven't
seen for a while. Arrange these in the front of your closet. Pack,

return, give, or throw away any maternity clothes that you are no longer wearing.

Returning to work is a stickier situation. You don't want to find out you have nothing to wear the night before you go back to work. Give yourself options. Put together a week's worth of outfits from your early pregnancy clothes. Do not even entertain the idea of wearing your maternity clothes. No matter what you think now, you will never again want to wear what you have been wearing for the last three to six months—or at least not for a long while. Another idea: borrow one or two outfits from a friend who is a little larger than your pre-pregnancy size. Or go catalog shopping while feeding your babe in the wee hours.

Dressing at home for the first few months is pretty easy: whatever you have time to grab. You do want to have lots of tops that pull up or dresses with buttons or other easy access to the mammary fountain. The reality is, you change a lot. The little wonder spits, pees, and poops on you. Milk dribbles under your arm. Your own bodily secretions can be rather, let us say, ripe. It can be nearly impossible to find time to shower, so changing your top can be the only recourse. A quick way to freshen up your underarms, but not your breasts, is to wipe them with astringent (witch hazel is good or a scented variety) on a cotton pad. Also, scented powder can soothe heat flashes.

Sensual Ideas

Show off your body; pregnancy is beautiful. Wear a plunging neckline and bare your new cleavage. Short skirts, bare backs, bare shoulders, and manicured hands can help you look as glorious as you are.

Buy yourself something to wear that is truly beautiful and elegant and that you can continue to enjoy after the baby is here. If your feet haven't swollen, shoes are an easy choice. A leather purse in the fall, an antique silk shawl in the spring, cashmere-lined gloves in the winter, excellent walking shoes for the summer. Stick to small indulgences like a leather headband or extra thick cotton socks if spending money on yourself is impossible because of financial concerns.

Wear less makeup if your face or eyes are puffy. Buy a lip pencil or lipstick in a bold color and accentuate your mouth instead of your eyes or cheeks.

Treat yourself to more than one shower a day with a fragrant shower gel.

Band-Aids over protruding belly buttons can prevent irritation.

Above all, remember that you are divine, exquisite, superb—you are literally glowing with life. Flaunt it!

Resources:

Pregnancy Chic: The Fashion Survival Guide, by Cherie Serota and Jody Kozlow Gardner (Villard, 1998). Tips on dressing. Aimed more towards slim women.

Websites:

Japanese Weekend (especially their belly stretch jeans)
http://www.japaneseweekend.com

Showing @ PregnancyFashion.com (Portal to all sorts of maternity wear)
http://PregnancyFashion.com

Mothers Work
http://www.motherswork.com/HomeBrand.asp (lists all their brands)

Preparing for Birth

You'll Need:

Books about birth.

Perhaps a childbirth education class to inform you of your choices.

Your journal or paper, and a pen.

Input from other women.

When to Do It:

- From conception to several months before your due date. (Early is fine, later is ticklish because you never know when that new life is going to wiggle out.)

- When you are feeling overwhelmed by birthing choices, terrified by what could go wrong, or when you are convinced your baby will never, ever emerge.

- If you feel a burst of "nesting" energy but aren't quite in the shape to paint the house or wallpaper the dining room.

What Is It?

The best advice about birthing is in Polly Berrien Berends's book *Whole Child/Whole Parent:*

> To leave your house, you first head for the door. But suppose as you near the door you become more concerned with the door itself than with passing through it. (Oh, what a beautiful carved door!) Perhaps you fear that the door will not open or that you personally will not be able to open it. . . . As long as you remain fascinated with the door it is not possible to pass through the doorway.

Childbirth is the doorway too many of us get stuck in—spending our pregnancy worrying and obsessing about the pain and possible complications, instead of focusing on the fact we are becoming parents, that "delivery is not a matter of expulsion but of revelation, since what is essentially happening for both ourselves and our babies is the further coming to light of what we already truly are."

That said, preparation for birth *is* necessary, because although it is far from the final destination, it *is* a very big, imposing doorway and the most dramatic and mysterious part of this mighty rite of passage. Unfortunately, it has become an overmedicated and romanticized passage. Your choices seem to be either have a C-section or have a religious experience. Deciding what would make your birth experience self-affirming and deciding you deserve such an experience can lead you to make the choices and get the education you need to guide your baby into the world in a joyful, peaceful way. It will also enhance your self-esteem as a mother and allow plenty of room for variation and change.

What to Do:

Envision Your Ideal Labor and Birth

What would your ideal pregnancy and birth experience be like? Being able to imagine the widest and best possibilities enlarges your choices. Consider this story from Basque anthropologist Angeles Arrien as told in *Bonding Before Birth* by Leni Schwartz:

> The Basque people of Spain treasure birth and their customs honor it as "a sacred art." Traditionally, Basque couples wait until they are in their 30s or 40s to have their families, feeling they are more mature. . . . The entire extended family gathers at the birth, including siblings, aunts, uncles, grandparents. All are considered birth attendants. The environment is carefully considered and when weather permits, the birth takes place out of doors, often near a running stream. There is a merry accompaniment of music: singing, chanting, drums, and flutes, plus storytelling and jokes to cheer the laboring mother. They speak of massaging the mother and baby with laughter. All the family stay together for seven days—and at the end of the ritual week celebrate with the entire village.

Let this story tickle your imagination to write a brief narrative of your ideal labor and birth. Don't let reality stop you; your imagination is the only limit. You can be an ancient Goddess or return to your ancestral land to be surrounded by extended family and ancient custom. Or you can live on Star Trek's *Enterprise* and have your baby beamed out. Borrow from anything and anyone. Is there something your sister had or did that you wish you could have or do? Put it in. If you are a single mother-to-be and wish you had a partner, let yourself have one. If you do have a partner but he or she is less than supportive, this is your chance to be clear about what you want. Maybe you see yourself being transformed by this experience, having angels help you, having God's hand brush you as you give birth? Focus on what *you* want. A good question to keep in mind while weaving your fantasy is "What activities, support, or birthing choices would enhance my self-esteem as a mother?" Don't concern yourself with spelling or making sense; this is for your eyes only!

Set this story aside for now; we'll come back to it later.

Educate Yourself

Birth has become a very well documented event. There is plenty of material available for you to peruse. As you explore various ideas, keep in mind the question "What kind of birth would enhance my self-esteem as a mother?" This question acts as a lightning rod to attract the information and support people that will help you make your birth as nurturing as possible.

See Resources for books on birthing.

Read up on various kinds of birthing practices. This will give you a much clearer idea of the range of choices available to you as well as expose you to new ideas and issues you might not have considered.

Ask whomever you would like present at the birth (your partner or friend) to write or describe his or her wishes for an ideal labor and birth. Have your partner do this before he or she reads yours.

Talk to other women who have given birth. Ask them what they liked and what they regretted about their babies' births. Canvass strangers in the grocery store (this works best if they have a baby with them), third cousins twice removed, as well as immediate family and friends.

Don't make the mistake of making the same birth preparation your best friend did because this seems easy and familiar. Your labor and delivery will be as unique as you are. If you want a birth that enhances your sense of self, you must give it conscious thought. That doesn't mean you can't choose the same things your friend did. Nor does it mean nine months of obsessive research. Invent a happy medium.

Consider attending a childbirth education class. Before I became pregnant, I assumed if you wanted a "natural" childbirth your only choice was Lamaze. That isn't true. Other techniques are also available, including the Bradley method and eclectic methods that borrow from many birth philosophies. Research the classes available in your area by talking to your health care provider, calling the hospitals in your area, asking instructors of pregnancy fitness classes, baby supply stores, and maternity clothing stores, or contacting the National Association of Childbirth.

Be wary of picking up birth values that lock you into a rigid expectation of how your birth must unfold. Imagining only one way of giving birth and being accepting of only that way don't allow enough room for the uniqueness of birth. Keeping an open mind and becoming well informed about all possibilities and options is by far the best approach.

Of course, the type of health care provider you have chosen will greatly influence your birth. However, don't hesitate to change health care providers if you are learning that a different style of birth would be better for you. It is not uncommon for women to switch horses midstream. I did. You don't owe your health care provider a thing. You need to feel very confident and excited about your choice. Don't let a misplaced sense of loyalty keep you in a health care relationship you are not comfortable with.

See Finding a Great Health Care Provider.

Preparing for Surprises

Creating a vision of your labor and delivery must include looking at possible disappointments and changes in your expectations and plans.

Because birth is the ultimate metaphor for life (that is, completely unpredictable), it is actually reassuring to consider what you don't want to have happen. Why? Because it can help you take steps and make choices to prevent it from happening. Also, if you think "that could never happen to me," you will be doubly bamboozled if you end up with prolonged labor, a C-section, or other surprises. Pamela said, "Don't box yourself into only one vision of your birth. You need to be able to change in the moment. What I resented about my birth experience was not calling the shots myself." If you have considered other possibilities, you are more likely to be able to stay in control, even if things don't go the way you envisioned.

Consider how you can prepare to be flexible about your birth experience. Areas to consider are:

If you are planning a natural delivery, how will you feel if you ask for drugs or must be given them? Discuss this with your partner or birth support person. Are you opposed to using drugs? Think carefully about your reasons for not wanting them. Does it have more to do with others' opinions? Consider how your self-image is invested in not having drugs; will you consider yourself a failure or a bad mother if you ask for some? Learn about the different drugs and their positive as well as negative effects. I'm not working for a pharmaceutical company, but I do feel that too many women limit themselves by refusing the option of drugs, creating pressure on themselves to perform in labor without taking into account how they may feel at that time and all the variables of birth. Having drugs during labor is just one of the many, many choices you must make as a parent.

What will you do if you have a C-section? Can you accept that as a possibility? What will it do to your self-image as a mother if you don't deliver vaginally?

What about the use of forceps or a vacuum extractor? How can you prepare to accept this as part of your birth experience if it must happen?

What happens if you end up needing bed rest? What would it be like for you to have to remain in bed for weeks?

If you are planning a home birth or to deliver at a free-standing birth center, what if you must transfer to the hospital? How can you prepare yourself emotionally for that alternative? What can you do to make it feel safe? Will you view it as a failure?

Many women I interviewed talked about how they had never considered any alternative to their ideal labor and delivery. Sometimes this is due to books and childbirth education classes that euphemistically describe labor pain as "discomfort" or "cramps." Be sure to learn about drugs, C-sections, and other choices and possibilities, and discuss them with your health care provider and birth partner. In the long run, confronting what you don't want is much more comforting than ignoring it.

Believing You Deserve It

Although no one can control birth, you can influence it. One of the most profound ways you can do that is to believe you deserve the birth you want. Read over the ideal labor and birth story that you recently wrote. As you read it, eavesdrop on what your internal critical voice is saying about your story. Quickly, without thinking, jot down what this voice is muttering to you.

An example:

Ideal labor and birth: My labor starts in the early afternoon. I feel a tremendous rush of energy, but I stay calm. I am able to do some painting in the early stages; I feel very creative, very alive, excited. Slowly, I get more and more crampy. By the time I need to start focusing on the contractions, I would already be five centimeters dilated. Jerry gets us ready to go to the hospital, but before we go, we walk up and down our road and watch a beautiful sunset.

At the hospital, I labor without drugs. It is very peaceful and private. I'm surrounded by pictures of home, my quilt, and other familiar things. I take several showers. I eat frozen yogurt and energy drinks. There is no need for an internal fetal monitor, and when the nurse does monitor me externally, she does so without being intrusive. Jerry and I communicate perfectly. He rubs my shoulders and stays close by at all times. I am able to walk around. No one tells me what to do. When I think I can't go on anymore, I am fully dilated and able to push. I am able to birth in whatever position I feel instinctively is best. I don't tear. I lift my baby to my chest. We are left alone, with Jerry, for an hour. Our baby is beautiful and perfect. When she is on my chest, all my fears about being a mom disappear. I have never felt better.

Critical voice is saying: You have never felt better. Ha! You'll be exhausted and screaming for drugs. You think you'll have this soft, lovely birth. Why should you give birth so perfectly? What makes you so special and different? People need to tell you what to do for your own good. You don't know better than the doctor. Anyway, birth is supposed to hurt. Why should you get out of it?

Take time to investigate and work with your critical voice. Ask yourself:

- Where did I learn these beliefs or feelings?

- What am I getting out of believing or feeling this way?

- Am I honestly willing to change these beliefs?

- What actions could I take to make my childbirth more nurturing?

An example: "You have never felt better. Ha! You'll be exhausted and screaming for drugs."

Where did I learn this belief? When I broke my arm, I couldn't stand the pain and made a fool out of myself begging for drugs. I felt bad because my mother always had such a high pain threshold and I was made to feel like a sissy if I cried when I got hurt.

What am I getting out of feeling this way? I can beat myself up later for failing to be tough.

Am I honestly willing to change this belief? Maybe I don't want to be tough. I don't want to feel pain. I'm just not willing to tough it out.

What actions could I take to make my childbirth more nurturing? I'll find out what the drugs do to the baby. I'll find out about other ways to manage pain, including visualization, hypnosis, and acupressure. I'll try to separate what my friends have told me I must do (natural child-birth) and what I want.

Another example: "Why should your birth be so special? What makes you so special and different?"

Where did I learn this belief? In grade school. I was told I was special at home but didn't find that reinforced in the world. I can especially remember Mrs. Miller's mean face saying I wasn't allowed to do something because I wasn't any different than the rest of the kids.

What am I getting out of feeling this way? I feel safe but depressed. I don't speak up for myself for fear of looking like I believe I'm special.

Am I honestly willing to change this belief? My baby's birth is the perfect place to say "Yes, I *am* special!"

What actions could I take to make my childbirth more nurturing? Taking the time and energy to visualize my giving birth. Doing special, self-nurturing things for myself *every day*. When I think about something special I want for my birth, like the birthing suite with the Jacuzzi, and I catch myself thinking I don't deserve it, sitting down and exploring that belief, trying to replace it with the feeling I do.

See Nurturing Yourself During Pregnancy: Giving Yourself Permission to Be Good to Yourself for a dialoguing technique that can be helpful in believing you deserve a wonderful birth.

The Ultimate Opportunity to Love Ourselves

What if instead of trying to prove something about ourselves during childbirth, demanding from ourselves that we perform perfectly, we viewed giving birth as an awesome chance to love ourselves, a chance to embrace who we are and let whatever happens be okay? Forget trying to control birth and judging ourselves for failing: "Well, I remembered the low moan but I still asked for drugs. It wasn't perfect." Here is a chance instead to "celebrate ourselves for our courage to birth. The real question becomes not, 'Have you done your breathing exercises?' but rather 'Can you love yourself no matter how you birth, where you birth, or what the outcome?'" writes Claudia Panuthos in her book, *Transformation through Birth.*

It is so important to go into your labor with your self-esteem high and the strength of conviction that "I can do this! My body knows how to do this!" That doesn't mean things won't change, nor does it mean there is only one acceptable style of birth. Work on *accepting yourself as you are now.* That is the foundation you want to labor from. From there, labor, no matter how it unfolds, will be exactly right.

Read over your ideal labor and birth story one more time. Does your story embrace yourself as you are now, or does it require you to be a little more perfect, strong, or stoic? This is not to say stretching yourself during labor is bad; in fact, it is almost always required. But there is always that fine line between stretching and never being enough, never accepting yourself. Which is it for you?

Also, as you read your story, are you willing to release this fantasy and accept whatever happens in its place? This doesn't mean you let your birth passively happen. You decide what you want and take realistic steps to make it happen. Then you let go. You can try hard and with the fierce intention to succeed, but you are able to accept a change in direction, able to accept the mystery of birth, without judging yourself a failure. One of the central spiritual lessons of birth is accepting that life is unpredictable and we are not in control. Another is it cannot be done perfectly. Accepting that can be a deeply enriching act of self-love.

Resources:

Birth as an American Rite of Passage, by Robbie Davis-Floyd (University of California Press, 1993). Fascinating interviews with 100 white middle-class women about their choices and birth experiences. Ms. Davis-Floyd is a cultural anthropologist, and her findings are stunning.

Birth Stories, by Jane Dwinell, R.N. (Bergin & Garvey, 1992). If you think reading other women's stories will help you prepare, this is a good selection.

Birthing from Within: An Extra-Ordinary Guide to Childbirth Preparation, by Pam England (Partera Press, 1998). One of the best books on preparing for birth. Filled with exercises to contact your feelings and body.

Getting Pregnant & Staying Pregnant: Overcoming Infertility and Managing Your High-Risk Pregnancy, by Diana Raab, Anita Levine-Goldberg, and Harry Farb (Hunter House, 1999). A judicious guide to the physical, medical, and emotional issues women, and their partners, face during infertility treatments and high-risk pregnancies.

Ina May's Guide to Childbirth, by Ina May Gaskin (Bantam, 2003). A comfortable and supportive read to support your body in what it does naturally. Alternative approach.

International Childbirth Education Association, P.O. Box 20048, Minneapolis, MN 55420-0048. Phone 612-854-8660 for information about childbirth educators in your area or visit http://www.icea.org.

Misconceptions: Truth, Lies, and the Unexpected on the Journey to Motherhood, by Naomi Wolf (Anchor, 2003). This book is NOT for the faint of heart. I admire Wolf for her unflinching honesty but wonder about her ability to be unbaised. Best bet if you are need help preparing for standing up for yourself in a less than ideal birth situation, especially in the United States.

Relax & Enjoy Your Baby: A Complete Program of Relaxation for New and Expectant Parents (two cassettes, 5, 10 and 15 min. segments) by Sylvia Klein Oklin, M.S. Helps mom and dad relax during pregnancy and early parenthood. Includes music by Bach, Vivaldi and Mozart, coupled with sounds of water and birds. 1–800–788–6670 or 516–621–2727

Special Deliverease™—Developed in partnership with a leading OB/Gyn, this comfort kit is a laboring woman's best friend. Filled with tools and treats for the birthing process. Find out where to buy at http://www.fortyweeks.com

The Unofficial Guide to Having a Baby, by Ann Douglas, John R. Sussman M.D. (John Wiley and Sons, 2004). A week-by-week guide to what's going on with your body, what's going on with your baby, and what's going on with your head for each of the forty weeks of pregnancy.

Whole Child/Whole Parent, by Polly Berrien Berends (Perennial, 1997). The classic text on the spiritual and creative life of children. Wonderful and practical.

Websites:

Doulas of North America
1–888–788-DONA
http://www.dona.org

International Childbirth Education Association, Inc.
http://www.icea.org

Surrender

Your journal and a
pen.

Large drawing paper
and paint, pencils,
or watercolors.

When to Do It

- If you refuse to acknowledge your life is changing.

- When you are terrified of any aspect of your pregnancy, especially
  childbirth.

- If you feel pregnancy has a spiritual component.

What Is It?

Surrender is the current running throughout pregnancy, labor, delivery, and most definitely into parenting. You surrender your body to the tiny being inside you, you surrender any garments with waists, you surrender to the pain of birth, you surrender to the sweet chaos of the early months of mothering.

The kind of surrender involved in pregnancy can best be described by an image of a fast-flowing river strewn with rocks. Imagine you are the water. You can choose to force yourself over the rocks, or you can flow around them. It might mean breaking into many streams or taking a number of detours, including detours into stagnant backwaters, but going with the flow of the river allows you to feel the life force sweeping through you. "Surrender involves letting go—of what we already know or have—and letting be—opening to the situations that life presents," writes clinical psychologist John Welwood in *Journey of the Heart*. Life is presenting you with a situation that involves asking for support and reassurance, surrendering expectations, opening to trust. This doesn't mean ignoring or downplaying your anger, resentment, and other mixed feelings. But no matter how much we learn or how much we fight, there are times when life requires us to soften and open, and pregnancy is one of the most poignant and instructive.

What to Do:

Write About It

Free-associate with the words *surrender, submit, go with the flow.* Do
this by writing whatever comes up without stopping to think or edit.
Commit to writing for *ten* minutes, keep your hand moving even when
you want to quit. Read what you've written. What can you gather from
your associations? Are there any insights you would like to build on,
actions you would like to take? Susan saw that she needed to work on
relaxing, so she decided to get a regular massage, listen to a relaxation
tape before bed, and to try and let little things go (like having the bed
perfectly made or her nails done). Sandra found images of water coming up as she wrote. She decided to spend several weekends alone at
the beach, contemplating the waves. "As I walked the beach, I just
kept thinking—no it was less thinking and more feeling—'go with the
flow.' I feel like it was my body rehearsing for labor."

Draw It

Draw what surrender looks like to you. Stay away from representational forms and try to express yourself in colors or abstract forms. To
get beyond the obvious, it helps to work with large paper and to do
several drawings.

Practice

Practice surrendering in little ways. During an orgasm is a good
opportunity—give yourself up to it. Perhaps you will feel an edge of
fear, the fear of being swept away, annihilated. Practice going beyond
that edge, surrendering a little more to the sensation.

Morning sickness can also present a strange opportunity to surrender.
Instead of pushing the sickness away, go toward it. Relinquish your
control. Go deeper into the nausea. (This sounds very weird and hard
to believe; experiment.)

You've Done It Before

Recall a time in which you let go and everything fell into place—a time when you stopped striving, when you sensed a power greater than yourself ordering your life, or when you stopped beating your head against the wall and listened instead to your inner voices of guidance and support or the advice of a respected friend. (If you can't think of such an incident, invent one.)

What Do You Need to Surrender?

What do you imagine yourself needing to surrender to during your pregnancy, labor, and after you have the child? Make three lists. Here are examples:

During Pregnancy

- Not being able to run in the marathon

- Having to go to the bathroom every fifteen minutes

- Going to bed at nine P.M.; slowing down in general

During Labor

- Letting go of having my baby safe inside me; fear of separation

- Wanting to run away from the pain; stop labor and quit

- A C-section if anything goes wrong

After the Baby Is Born

- Being interrupted when I want to read and write in my journal

- Feeling tugged in two different directions when I go back to work

- Sex with my partner without planning and effort

See the rituals in Ambivalence: Grieving the Changes.

Acknowledging the change that is taking place can help you begin to let go. Sometimes that is enough. If making this list doesn't feel sufficient, do a ritual around grieving.

Spiritual Surrender

If you can, imagine yourself offering your gas pains, your exhaustion, your fears, your nausea to your God, Goddess, Higher Power, or the Earth. Aloud, say, "I surrender this to you." Give it up. Stop struggling alone.

Create your own simple meditation to help you yield and let go. Mine was a walking incantation: "Softly open, gratefully joyous." I would recite this as I walked down a beautiful lane, through a patch of woods, across Mission Creek, and up steep steps to a stone shrine of the Virgin Mary. I would pray or just allow myself to be. Then back home repeating with each step, "Softly open, gratefully joyous."

Postpartum

One friend practices surrender with her newborn by reacting to each minidisaster or distraction or detour with a silent prayer, "I surrender." When she is talking on the phone and he awakens early she can get tense—"I expected more time to talk"—or she can say, "I surrender." (And she can also silently call him several choice names.)

Surrendering to motherhood is done in stages. Each new stage of growth brings a new level of surrender, a renewed struggle for patience, a deeper level of acceptance and enjoyment. You recommit each day to being a mother.

Resources:

Start Where You Are A Guide to Compassionate Living, by Pema Chodron (Shambhala, 2001). No need to wait for things to change to start creating more inner peace and wisdom.

Meditation Secrets for Women: Discovering Your Passion, Pleasure, and Inner Peace, by Camille Maurine and Lorin Roche (HarperSanFrancisco, 2001). An encyclopedia of feminine and body centered ways to meditate. If you've always thought meditation meant sitting still or following a guru, you need this book.

Comfort at a Glance

	INTRODUCTION	NURTURING YOURSELF DURING PREGNANCY	A PREGNANCY JOURNAL	HOW TO GRACEFULLY ASK FOR AND ACCEPT SUPPORT	FORMING YOUR SUPPORT TEAM	FINDING A GREAT HEALTH CARE PROVIDER	I AM A BODY WITHOUT A BRAIN	AM I FAT AND UGLY OR ROUND AND BEAUTIFUL?	TUMULTUOUS, TURBULENT FEELINGS	CONNECTING WITH YOUR PARTNER	IT'S NOT ALL IN YOUR HEAD: SURVIVING THE PHYSICAL DISCOMFORT OF PREGNANCY	FOOD	COMFORTING CLOTHING AND OTHER SENSUAL STRATEGIES	PREPARING FOR BIRTH	SURRENDER
Adjusting Postbaby	3	19			32	48	52		69	76			117		133
Afraid of Becoming My Mother															130
Afraid of My Relationship Suffering								61	71	75					
Agog with It All			23				52		67						
Allowing Support In	6		26	28	36				69	79	91	109		121	130
Allowing Yourself to Be Dependent	3	11		30						87	94				130
Ambivalent	4								73	78	100				
Anger	3	17					51		67		89				
Anxiety	6	18								86				123	130
Baby's Nap Time		19							69						
Balance	3	10							71				105		
Becoming a Stay-at-Home Mom	3									82					
Birth Options						44							117	120	
Birth Support		11		30		47							117	122	
Boring Maternity Clothes	4				36								111		
Breast-Feeding (or Not)															
Bursting with Joy		18	26				56	63					117		133
Can't Take Time for Self	3	14			36		51	64	69		94	103			
Cesarean										86				123	132
Child Care															
Constipated											97				
Crave Beauty							55						118		
Craving Comfort Food												103			
Depressed									57	72	86				
Don't Want to Do Anything		12	24				53			72					130
Eating Habits												102			
Emotional Growth	5	14	24	28	33		53	57	67			107		125	130
Exercise								63			95				

AMBIVALENCE: GRIEVING THE CHANGES	FEAR	WORK	I WANT MY MOMMY	THE POETIC SIDE OF PREGNANCY: CREATIVITY, DREAMS, AND THE NEED FOR BEAUTY	THE SPIRITUAL SUSTENANCE OF PREGNANCY	WHAT'S GOING TO HAPPEN TO ME AFTER THE BABY IS BORN?	PREPARING FOR POSTPARTUM	A BABY AND MOTHER BLESSING JOURNEY	POSTBIRTH NOURISHMENT: SURVIVING AND THRIVING	POSTBIRTH NOURISHMENT: SURVIVING THE EMOTIONS	RECEIVING THE NURTURING YOU NEED FROM YOUR PARTNER POSTPARTUM (AND GIVING A LITTLE TOO)	BUT ISN'T SELF-NURTURING IMPOSSIBLE WITH INFANTS AND TODDLERS?	FINAL NOTES	APPENDIX: HERBS, OILS, AND OTHER NATURAL COMFORTERS	
143	148	163	179			203	209		231	252		292	305	314	Adjusting Postbaby
	155		175			200					278				Afraid of Becoming My Mother
141															Afraid of My Relationship Suffering
				183	191	203		223							Agog with It All
		164	179	186	195		211	223					305		Allowing Support In
			171		196			223			282		305		Allowing Yourself to Be Dependent
140	154	162			195	205				263		299			Ambivalent
141	148	164	176						243	261	277	299			Anger
	148		179	184	195			223		261					Anxiety
					198				247			297			Baby's Nap Time
		164	173	187	198		209		252	275			305		Balance
	168		176			205					284	296			Becoming a Stay-at-Home Mom
	152			187											Birth Options
	152				98			223	234						Birth Support
															Boring Maternity Clothes
							214		238		280			314	Breast-Feeding (or Not)
			179	184	194	203	210	223	234	261	282		305		Bursting with Joy
		159	171	189	198		211	223	239	268	283	292	305		Can't Take Time for Self
									243						Cesarean
		165	179				217			268	285	298			Child Care
															Constipated
			179	183	193	203		223							Crave Beauty
			171							237					Craving Comfort Food
142	148		171	183	195	203	218		231	270				309	Depressed
			171												Don't Want to Do Anything
									233						Eating Habits
141	147		176	187	195	200			246	252		303			Emotional Growth
					191				234	255					Exercise

Comfort at a Glance

	Introduction	Nurturing Yourself During Pregnancy	A Pregnancy Journal	How to Gracefully Ask For and Accept Support	Forming Your Support Team	Finding a Great Health Care Provider	I Am a Body Without a Brain	Am I Fat and Ugly or Round and Beautiful?	Tumultuous, Turbulent Feelings	Connecting With Your Partner	It's Not All in Your Head: Surviving the Physical Discomfort of Pregnancy	Food	Comforting Clothing and Other Sensual Strategies	Preparing for Birth	Surrender
Fear of Being an Inadequate Mother	5	15							71	86	91			126	
Fear of Losing My Identity		18	25					59		86					
Feel Like an Ugly Whale							55	57				104	111		
Feeling the Creative Urge		18			36			60				106		121	131
Fighting the Changes				28			53	59	70	76					130
Finding a Pediatrician						48									
Finding Support	6					43				81					
Friendship	6			30	32										
Gas												97			133
Gatekeeping															
Grasping the Enormity		10	23				53								
Grieving	4										91				
Guilt		17					54		71		89		101		
Harsh Expectations for Partner						47				81					
Harsh Expectations for Self		14		28			54	60	71	81	90			123	
Hate My Doctor				34		43					91			123	
Having Sex Again															
Herpes															
How to Eat												92	100		
I'm Open Wide	3	11					56		67						
Including Your Partner			26	30	40	47		61		75		94			
Insomnia												96			
Intrusive Family					38	47				83					132
Keeping Up at Work		18											118		
Lonely				30	35					75					
Loving Your Body	3						55	57					118		
Lustful		13								84					
Memory Loss			24	28			52								
Miss My Java												103			
Money										86			118		
Mood Swings	3	10						60	67	81					131

Comfort at a Glance

AMBIVALENCE: GRIEVING THE CHANGES	FEAR	WORK	I WANT MY MOMMY	THE POETIC SIDE OF PREGNANCY: CREATIVITY, DREAMS, AND THE NEED FOR BEAUTY	THE SPIRITUAL SUSTENANCE OF PREGNANCY	WHAT'S GOING TO HAPPEN TO ME AFTER THE BABY IS BORN?	PREPARING FOR POSTPARTUM	A BABY AND MOTHER BLESSING JOURNEY	POSTBIRTH NOURISHMENT: SURVIVING AND THRIVING	POSTBIRTH NOURISHMENT: SURVIVING THE EMOTIONS	RECEIVING THE NURTURING YOU NEED FROM YOUR PARTNER POSTPARTUM (AND GIVING A LITTLE TOO)	BUT ISN'T SELF-NURTURING IMPOSSIBLE WITH INFANTS AND TODDLERS?	FINAL NOTES	APPENDIX: HERBS, OILS, AND OTHER NATURAL COMFORTERS	
142	154	163	171	187	197	205	211	223		258	279	292	305	309	Fear of Being an Inadequate Mother
142	156	162	175	187		200			236			300		309	Fear of Losing My Identity
			179	187	193		213		233	266					Feel Like an Ugly Whale
143				183	193	203		223							Feeling the Creative Urge
142	148	159		187		200	209	223		260					Fighting the Changes
											280				Finding a Pediatrician
		164	180				216			271					Finding Support
		164					216	223	236		277				Friendship
															Gas
			180				217				278	298			Gatekeeping
				187	195		209	223	234				305		Grasping the Enormity
143			178			204			238	263					Grieving
142		163				205			244	258	279	293			Guilt
142		166					211		244						Harsh Expectations for Partner
142	151	163	176	187	191	205	211		249	258	279	293	305		Harsh Expectations for Self
															Hate My Doctor
											288				Having Sex Again
														312	Herpes
										255					How to Eat
142	148				197					257			305		I'm Open Wide
145	151	166		186	197		211		240	269	275	298			Including Your Partner
										260				312	Insomnia
			180		197						277				Intrusive Family
		159										296			Keeping Up at Work
142			179	183			219	223		265					Lonely
			179	187	191					266					Loving Your Body
									241		290				Lustful
									247	259					Memory Loss
														307	Miss My Java
		169	173									295			Money
142			171						231	252			305	309	Mood Swings

Comfort at a Glance

	INTRODUCTION	NURTURING YOURSELF DURING PREGNANCY	A PREGNANCY JOURNAL	HOW TO GRACEFULLY ASK FOR AND ACCEPT SUPPORT	FORMING YOUR SUPPORT TEAM	FINDING A GREAT HEALTH CARE PROVIDER	I AM A BODY WITHOUT A BRAIN	AM I FAT AND UGLY OR ROUND AND BEAUTIFUL?	TUMULTUOUS, TURBULENT FEELINGS	CONNECTING WITH YOUR PARTNER	IT'S NOT ALL IN YOUR HEAD: SURVIVING THE PHYSICAL DISCOMFORT OF PREGNANCY	FOOD	COMFORTING CLOTHING AND OTHER SENSUAL STRATEGIES	PREPARING FOR BIRTH	SURRENDER
Mothering the Mother	3	14		28	35		56		73	86		105	117	121	
Moving				28	32	43									
Nauseated		17					54	66	73	84	90				131
Needy		11		30				62	70	87					
Overwhelmed	5		23		39		51		68	82	91	100	112		130
Panic Attacks							54		72	86					
Partner Is a Woman		9			36			63	73	80					
Perfection Monster	2	14		28			53		73		89	100		125	130
Permission to Be Good to Yourself	4	14		28			55	57	72			103	118	125	130
Powerful Dreams										79					
Pregnant Pleasures		18			33		51	63		76		103	118		
Regretful		15							68					124	130
Resentful		15			38			60	68						130
Ritual		15	26				55	63		87		102			133
Sad	4	15		28				59	68						
Selfish	2	11		28					87	95					
Setting Boundaries		16			39	44			69		95	103		127	
Sex									84						131
Single Mom		9		29	45				73	75	90			122	
Sleep Deprivation									83	96					133
Spiritually Yearning			26	28			51	63						122	133
Survival		16		28			52		67	83	90	108		120	
Terrified of Labor		10				43			79					120	131
Terrified of Losing the Baby										86					130
Time Monster		8	24				54					106	113		130
Too Old to Be Pregnant		9							73						
Unsupportive Partner		9		29	33			61		77	90			122	
Veteran Mom		9	24	28	32				69	75	95				
Why Caring for Yourself Is Good for Your Child				28			56					103			
Witching Hour							52								133
Work		16							71				118		
Worn Out	3	16		28			53	63			94	103			133

AMBIVALENCE: GRIEVING THE CHANGES	FEAR	WORK	I WANT MY MOMMY	THE POETIC SIDE OF PREGNANCY: CREATIVITY, DREAMS, AND THE NEED FOR BEAUTY	THE SPIRITUAL SUSTENANCE OF PREGNANCY	WHAT'S GOING TO HAPPEN TO ME AFTER THE BABY IS BORN?	PREPARING FOR POSTPARTUM	A BABY AND MOTHER BLESSING JOURNEY	POSTBIRTH NOURISHMENT: SURVIVING AND THRIVING	POSTBIRTH NOURISHMENT: SURVIVING THE EMOTIONS	RECEIVING THE NURTURING YOU NEED FROM YOUR PARTNER POSTPARTUM (AND GIVING A LITTLE TOO)	BUT ISN'T SELF-NURTURING IMPOSSIBLE WITH INFANTS AND TODDLERS?	FINAL NOTES	APPENDIX: HERBS, OILS, AND OTHER NATURAL COMFORTERS	
143		164	171	183	199	200	209	223	231	252	277	292	305	306	Mothering the Mother
				185											Moving
142	147													308	Nauseated
142			171			203	217	223	240	256	282	292		309	Needy
143	148	159	179	189	198	200	216		232	257		292			Overwhelmed
142	148		179							261				309	Panic Attacks
		161									276				Partner Is a Woman
	151	163	178		195	205	211		232			293	305		Perfection Monster
		164	173		191	203	209	223	231	253	283	292	305		Permission to Be Good to Yourself
				185		200			234						Powerful Dreams
145			179	183	193	203		223							Pregnant Pleasures
140			177			200				263	281				Regretful
140		162	174			205	221		231	264	282	299			Resentful
142	153		179	187	195	204		223	234		281				Ritual
142			175			205			238		281			309	Sad
		162		187	197	200	209		240	252		292			Selfish
		164	180			207	217		247	268	277	294			Setting Boundaries
											288				Sex
145	155	161	173			200	217	223			275	293			Single Mom
142			181						243	269	278			307	Sleep Deprivation
143	153		172	183	191	204		223	234						Spiritually Yearning
		164					209		231	252	277	292			Survival
142	150			189				223						309	Terrified of Labor
142	149				195					259				309	Terrified of Losing the Baby
		163							246	258		297			Time Monster
143	155														Too Old to Be Pregnant
142	155		171		195		217	223							Unsupportive Partner
140	150	163	180	184		201	209		235		286	293			Veteran Mom
						205			231	253	277	303	305		Why Caring for Yourself Is Good for Your Child
	148										284				Witching Hour
		157	173		195		221		241	268		296			Work
	148	163	171		199		216		235	258	287	292		307	Worn Out

Ambivalence

Grieving the Changes

You'll Need:

A few uninterrupted minutes alone.

Two candles.

A timer.

When to Do It:

- If in early pregnancy, you find yourself cursing the tadpole in your belly because you are sick or in shock or things just aren't going the way you envisioned.

- If you are afraid your mate will love the baby more than you.

- If you've been having fantasies of flying to Fiji and somehow leaving your uterus behind.

- When you have decided to quit your job, move to a new community, buy or sell your house, or otherwise uproot your life even more.

- When you already have one or more children.

- If you have already had your baby and are astonished at your feelings.

What Is It?

At first, it may sound weird to link grieving with pregnancy. As you make the transition into motherhood, you may want to focus solely on what is beginning, not what is ending. And while that may sound optimistic and healthy, it sets up the belief that this new experience must only be positive. It leaves no room for the big A: ambivalence. Ambivalence is the coexisting of mutually conflicting feelings, such as love and hate. *The most universal feeling during pregnancy among women*

I interviewed was ambivalence. Don't feel shocked or gypped because you aren't blissed out every moment of your pregnancy. It is completely natural to feel conflicted over having a baby, to feel so sick that you wish you weren't pregnant, to chafe over what you will be giving up. Pregnancy is an emotionally challenging time, and almost every woman experiences unpleasant feelings. The problem arises when you don't let yourself grieve the change, when you focus only on "getting the baby" as family therapist Laura Evans says, and ignore the importance of saying good-bye to parts of your present identity, whether that identity includes you as a childless woman or as the mother of one child or as part of a couple.

Having a child stirs up a host of mixed feelings: excitement over creating a family and fear your relationship with your partner will be hurt; awe over the miracle of life and sadness at having to share your time; pride at your body carrying a child and anger over your changing body; pleasure at the thought of staying home and panic at giving up your adult life. For women who have struggled to become pregnant or waited until just the right moment, feeling ambivalent can be especially surprising and frightening. "I've chosen this. I want it. That means it can only be a good thing."

If you try to discuss your mixed feelings, friends may say, "Don't worry. You'll be a great mother" or "You'll be able to find plenty of time for your first child" or "You'll love that baby so much, it won't matter." All of these things might be true, but it doesn't change how you feel. These cheery statements can make you feel even more depraved.

Grieving for aspects of your life that are going to change (or if you read this postpartum, have changed) is not irreverent or melodramatic. By exploring and releasing your regrets, doubts, and anger over being pregnant or having the child, you can put your ambivalence into perspective and see life as it is: constant change where little is black or white. Your ambivalence won't go away (motherhood is a very dualistic reality), but it won't overwhelm you; you won't have to put energy into fighting it or into feeling guilty. If you can acknowledge the sorrow inherent in such gargantuan change, you open the door to a richer, more joyous, less conflicted view of your new role. You can love being a mother and hate it in the same moment, and that's okay. But if you deny your sadness, anger, or misgivings, you dampen your ability to feel the good stuff too. Also, a chunk of the conflict that results in postpartum shock and sometimes depression is not accepting the natural ambivalence you may be feeling.

Grieving doesn't mean your life will be terrible with a baby. *Not at all*. But by recognizing what you *fear* losing, what you may resent, you can adjust to your life with baby faster and with less baby shock. If you spend a few minutes now grieving for losses and changes that don't materialize, you will be that much more appreciative and aware. This applies to postpartum as well. Grieving for what seems terrible or sad or irretrievable in the moment doesn't mean it won't seem better in a few days or even minutes. It also doesn't mean you shouldn't grieve for how you feel right now.

What to Do:

Each of these simple rituals can be combined and/or done more than once, and they are especially effective after the baby arrives. They work best if you are relaxed, alone, and uninterrupted. Each ritual can be done in five to ten minutes.

Bubble Visualization

This ritual can be more powerful with melancholy or angry music, depending upon your mood.

Close your eyes. Imagine yourself enshrined in a bubble. This bubble looks however you choose, but it is big enough to hold you inside. Within the bubble you can say or do *anything* without hurting *anyone*. It can contain all your feelings, no matter how strong. Envision yourself inside the bubble. Picture what the walls look and feel like. Test the walls to be sure you believe they are impregnable. When it feels safe, list everything that is bugging you, worrying you, making you testy, sad, out-of-sorts, gloomy, or causing you pain. Be specific. Be as graphic and honest as you can bear. As you speak, see the bubble absorb your words. Perhaps the wall of the bubble momentarily turns a different color as it absorbs your feelings. Or perhaps there is a sound of sizzling. Or a zap. Whatever you see or hear is perfect. When you have vented your feelings as thoroughly as you dare, unzip or puncture a hole in the bubble and step out; now visualize the bubble collapsing on itself like a deflating rubber beach ball until it is small enough to hold in your hand. Feel its weight. Visualize yourself disposing of the ball in whatever way feels good: throwing it over the moon and out into hyperspace, flying on the wind to Alaska and tucking it under a glacier, burning it in a volcano. Be sure you feel the bubble and all it holds is gone. If you don't, dispose of it again.

Candle Ritual

Create a sacred space by burning some incense, meditating for a few moments, or otherwise centering yourself. Place two candles in front of you. Light one. As you do so, recite: "As I light this candle, I remember the parts of my self and my life I fear losing after the baby is born. [If you are doing this postpartum, change to 'the parts of myself I feel I have lost.'] As I take a few moments to gaze at the flame, I review my life as it was before I became pregnant." Take a few minutes to reflect on your prebaby life. Forget chronological order or importance. I remembered carefree walks with my dog, month-long canoe trips, hours to read, time alone with Chris, time alone, period. I knew I would have these moments again, but I also knew they would be much less frequent and simply different. Give yourself permission to reflect and reminisce.

When you are ready, light the second candle by the flame of the first as you recite, "As I light this new candle, I celebrate the new life beginning for me and my baby. [If you are doing this postpartum, change to 'the new me and my new baby that has been born.'] As I take a few moments to gaze into this flame, I anticipate my life with this wondrous new person." Take another minute to envision your postbaby life. Again, anything goes—from foreseeing your baby's first smile to watching yourself saying just the right thing as you soothe her after her first broken heart.

Finally, blow out the first candle, saying, "Although this light is gone, and with it this stage of my life, the new flame sustains those parts of me and brings into light new parts. I bring all of me, perfect and imperfect, conflicted and happy, to my new role as mother of this child."

This ritual can also be done with a friend, partner, or group of new moms. Each person can take turns naming aloud what she or he is grieving for and celebrating. It takes quite a bit of trust to share this, but it can be very powerful.

Postpartum

If you are doing this ritual postpartum, you might want to consider the list of losses below as you grieve the parts of your life you have lost.

- spontaneity; freedom; being irresponsible

- self as an individual, only yourself to take care of; independence

- time alone; privacy

- career; money of your own

- sleep; energy; health

- confidence

- pregnancy; the child inside of you; the first step toward independence

- control over your life

- ability to complete tasks; ability to concentrate

- protection from dealing with early childhood issues

- friendships, especially with single or childless friends; feeling abandoned by family or friends

- being your mother or father's little girl

- your previous or desired physical shape; youth

- intimacy with partner or ability to date; not being married very long before childbirth

- identity as a sexual being

- adult company

- your fantasy of yourself as a perfect mother

- your fantasy of your child looking or acting a certain way

- your fantasy of your family looking or feeling a certain way

- the special attention that comes with being pregnant

- previous abortions or miscarriages

- single moms: grieving for the lack of help with pregnancy and baby

Which of these losses are you feeling? Read each one that fits you. Be still and allow yourself to feel that particular loss. If you start to feel overwhelmed, set a timer for two minutes. When the timer goes off, you are free not to feel or think about this.

It is completely natural to grieve the changes you are experiencing. Almost all mothers do. It is natural to grieve the addition of another child to your family, to grieve how much more complicated and hard two (or more) children are. It is completely natural to grieve your spontaneous free life and to wish you had waited a few more years. *None of this makes you a bad mother.* Don't waste energy blocking your sadness, fear, or shock. If possible, allow yourself daily, timed grieving sessions. Feel your sadness and move through it.

A Couple's Ritual

Together, pick a private and special place that represents your present relationship. A romantic camping spot, your own bed, a sweeping vista are possibilities. Separately, pick two small, inexpensive, or "found" gifts. One represents your life together so far. The second gift symbolizes your new life as parents and lovers.

Relax in your chosen spot. Take turns reminiscing about your life together. The focus does not need to be on activities that may be harder or impossible to do in the future. The point is to honor what you have shared, from late night bowling and mountain biking in Sri Lanka to a vegetable garden and finding the perfect sofa.

Next, take turns verbalizing what changes you fear the baby will bring to your relationship. Be as honest as you can. "I'm afraid you will love the baby more than me" or "I'm afraid we won't be able to handle the strain of raising a child together" or "I'm afraid of being too impatient, which you hate, and seeming ugly to you." Talking about your worries now can head off problems later. (If you are already parents, try to avoid talking about how the baby will affect your present child and stick to your relationship. Focus on the other child another time.)

When you feel you have talked enough, exchange your gifts. If necessary, explain to your partner what each symbolizes. For example, you might give your partner a piece of a battered bike chain to symbolize all the hundreds of miles you rode together, then a date book with "couple dates" already written in, starting eight weeks after the baby is due.

End by talking to your growing fetus. Explain to him you love him; tell her you welcome her, but you have been a couple alone so far and needed to make time to celebrate the past and recognize the change.

Resources:

Good Grief Rituals, by Elaine Childs-Gowell, A.R.N.P., Ph.D. (Station Hill, 1992). Although this book doesn't address pregnancy, it does talk about grieving for all sorts of events, from the death of a pet to betrayal by a friend. A wide range of rituals.

The Mask of Motherhood: How Becoming a Mother Changes Everything and Why We Pretend It Doesn't, by Susan Maushart (Penguin, 2000). Read this with care—some find it depressing, other liberating. Very helpful for older mothers.

Websites:

Hip Mama
http://www.hipmama.com

Fear

When to Do It:

- When you are walking by someone mowing a lawn, and you suddenly envision the mower going out of control and mowing you down. (Three women reported this nightmare.)

- If you've been feeling ill, and when you start to feel better you are sure you've lost the baby.

- When your mate is ten minutes late, you spend the entire time imagining the horrible car accident he is in and how you will manage as a single parent.

What Is It?

"Is the baby okay?" "Will I make it through labor?" "How will I get its tiny arms through the sleeves of its tiny outfits?" "What if I hate being a mother?" "What if something happens to my partner?" Dismaying possibilities, dreadful notions, horrible scenarios wake you at 3 A.M., dim your mind during a meeting, hinder you from becoming informed about labor and delivery, and nag you until your last good nerve is frayed. Fear is the shadow side of love, and love comes flooding into your life when you are pregnant. Pregnancy and motherhood bring an amplified sensitivity to the very real dangers in the world. You become more vulnerable to fears of the unknown. This is often coupled with an awakened awareness of hidden aspects of your unconscious, as new light is shone on previously unexamined areas. All together it can be a confusing, shocking, primitive experience. Perhaps this happens because of a mix of hormonal changes and the heightened awareness of the life cycle that comes from being close to

You'll Need:

A good childbirth education class.

Courage to question your health care provider and to talk about scary situations.

birth. But it does seem the more the fetus inside you becomes real, the more you see impending disaster everywhere (this is also true postpartum).

Acknowledging and working with your fears not only can make you feel more peaceful, but can help you have an easier labor—maybe not less painful, but definitely less overwhelming and frightening. Facing your fears can motivate you to change areas of your life you haven't paid enough attention to. Every pregnant woman and new mom experiences anxiety. *You can find comfort.*

What to Do:

Controlling Monkey Mind

Monkey mind describes what your mind is doing when it is caught up in worrying incessantly and imagining the worst. Your imagination is chasing its own tail, chattering about all the bad things that can happen, and you feel powerless to control it. Excellent comfort for monkey mind can be found by practicing this simple meditation. Next time you catch yourself frozen in terror over what you will wear to her Carnegie Hall debut (she'll be playing the piano and violin simultaneously), try these ideas:

Close your eyes. Visualize a circle with a line through it over your fearful scene. If, for example, you fear having a horrible labor, see your fearful version, then put a big red line through it, very emphatic. Now tune in to your body. Where does it feel tense? Perhaps your neck is tense or your stomach or forehead. Massage this tense area while inhaling deeply and saying silently, "I am at peace." Exhale by saying, "Mmmm," as if you're tasting something delicious. Repeat until you feel calm.

A related calming meditation practiced by Deb, a yoga instructor and mother of three, is to breathe a violet, cooling, healing mist into her fear. Start at your feet and imagine this soothing mist traveling up your body, inside and out. As you inhale this sweet, restorative mist, it relaxes all the parts of your body that are tight, rigid, fearful. As you exhale, let go of a little of the fear. Inhale the refreshing violet mist, focusing on feeling its healing in your physical self. Exhale your fear, your negative thoughts, your worries.

For particularly stubborn or disturbing thoughts (especially if you are experiencing obsessive thoughts postpartum), visualize the word STOP. Take a moment to decorate or dress each letter. You might draw leopard spots on the *S,* embroider the *T* with healing symbols, dress the *O* like Humpty Dumpty, and make the *P* into a bird that flies away.

Fears About the Baby's Health and Well-Being

Fears about the baby's health are the most frightening because they cannot be completely explained away. What helps?

Ask your health care provider, "What are the odds that my child will have anything wrong with him or her?" Be sure your health care provider is *specific.* Every word uttered on the subject of defects becomes etched in your mind. Get it straight and get reassurance or you may find yourself misinterpreting something he or she says and becoming even more afraid.

If you are worried, have an ultrasound. If you can't sleep, have an amniocentesis. But before you do, discuss with your partner, your spiritual mentor, or whomever feels appropriate what you will do if you discover something is wrong. Will you continue the pregnancy? How would you deal with a decision to abort? Will you have a funeral or some kind of ceremony if you do? Although this is very scary and depressing, sharing your fears with others can help you face them and wrap your mind around ways you would deal with the very worst case (and extraordinarily unlikely) scenario.

Photocopy a picture of a fetus in utero, or if you have one, use your ultrasound image. Post this where you can see it every day. When you see the image, put your hands on your belly and visualize your grow-ing baby listening to you as you say, "You are growing perfectly. You are whole and healthy. Everything is going to be perfect."

Educate yourself about what is happening in your body. Learn about the development of your baby at each stage. Check out *A Child Is Born,* Linnart Nilsson's classic pictorial of the growth of a fetus.

Someone told Diane when she was pregnant about a baby dying soon after birth. "It sent me to bed for three days. I let myself mope, I got into considering what that would be like. I thought through it, let myself be crazy." By confronting the worst and making a place for it in her mind, Diane was able to make a shakey peace with that possibility.

Fears About Labor and Delivery

Having a baby hurts. For some women, it will be the most painful experience of their lives. For others, it will hardly make an impression. First-time moms cannot truly grasp or fully prepare for labor because it is so entirely unknown. Veteran moms know each birth is different. One woman will tell you it feels like giving birth to a bowling ball. Another will say it felt like really bad cramps. You might meet someone who had three contractions and delivered. You keep saying to yourself, "How bad can it be?"

See Preparing for Birth.

Learn about *normal* birth. Watch videos of uncomplicated deliveries; you can borrow them from your health care provider, your hospital, a birth center, or a library. Jodie perused black-and-white photos of a friend's birth to help her visualize what birth looked like. Seek out positive, detailed birth stories from women who have recently given birth. This doesn't mean you shouldn't learn about C-sections, forceps, and vacuum extractors but that you should imagine yourself having the most normal delivery possible. Take a childbirth education class that emphasizes normal delivery but avoid classes that won't mention the word *pain*. You want a class that gives you concrete suggestions on how to deal with pain and complications (especially information about drugs and C-sections), that tells you what to expect from your recovery from complications, and that also reinforces the idea that you can *try* to create the birth you want.

On the other hand, it is not necessary to become an obstetrician to have a baby. You don't have to spend the next nine months reading every book and taking ten courses. Learning too much can sometimes be a handicap. If you know you will only freak yourself out more, take it easy on the scholarship.

The real event is helping your child grow up; the process of labor and birth is an infinitesimal part of being a parent. No matter how bad your labor is or how long it takes, it is only a fraction of your life.

Billions of women have done it.

It will end. It will not last forever.

Screen out birth stories told by women who seem to want to terrify you. Politely but firmly tell them something like, "I respect what a horrible time you had, but it makes me uncomfortable to hear that now." Some women will persist. Don't listen just to be polite! Remind yourself, *every woman's labor is different.*

If you are frightened of failing at birth, losing control, begging for drugs, or otherwise not fitting a preconceived expectation of the consummate woman giving birth, it is time to burn these concerns. *There is no perfect way to have a baby.* Although the concept of actively participating in the birth is a crucial one, it has been blown out of proportion. To actively participate does not mean you must control every aspect of yourself and your environment or you are a failure. Performance anxiety has become a real problem during labor. But labor is like mothering: you prepare and do the best you can, but finally, most of it is out of your hands. Birth is a great mystery. Yet we live in a rational, scientific world that doesn't allow for mystery. "In this day and age, there must be a better way to have a baby" implies that if you are informed enough, strong enough, you can control it. Any woman who has given birth, who can be honest, will tell you otherwise. There are no guarantees. It is an uncontrollable experience. Taking care of yourself and being informed and empowered are crucial, but so is surrender. Forget about trying to birth perfectly. Forget about trying to please anyone, least of all your doctor or midwife, and especially your mate.

See Preparing for Birth; and Surrender.

If you fear your mate cannot handle seeing you in pain or will freak out during labor, or you fear being embarrassed in front of him or her, tell your partner your fears. Use "I" statements so your mate doesn't feel blamed. "I am worried about how my being in pain may make

See Finding a Great Health Care Provider: The Magic of a Birth Support Person.

you feel. Can we talk about this?" Ask, "What are your fears during labor? What can I do to make this birth easier for you?" If necessary, have a session or two with a therapist to help you discuss the issue. You don't want to feel inhibited during birth; you want to feel safe and supported. Consider hiring a birth support person to take the pressure off your mate to perform.

Transforming Your Fears About Labor and Delivery

Visit where you will give birth. Visualize yourself in this setting. Notice the smells, the sounds, the sights. Does this place feel okay? What don't you like? At first, I planned to have Lillian at a birth center, but I discovered as I toured the rooms that I didn't feel comfortable. The staff was great, but I couldn't see myself giving birth there. Pay attention to your senses, your impressions, and especially your fears. Let them push you to be as persistent and assertive as you need to be to become reassured. Pregnancy is preparation for parenthood, where you must take responsibility. Take responsibility for yourself now as training. If you have any little fears, like not knowing where to park or how to use the controls on the bed or what it will feel like to have people coming in and out of your room, use this visit to ask *plenty* of detailed questions. This is the time to be assertive.

Take a few moments whenever you can (once or twice a week is excellent, but even once in your pregnancy is beneficial) visualizing yourself giving birth. Listen to a relaxation tape or soothing music until you feel like water running downhill—light and flowing. Picture yourself in the setting in which you will be giving birth. See your birth partner, your health care provider, and any other participants supporting and comforting you perfectly. See yourself handling the pain the way you would like. Be sure to visualize any particularly fearful situations going well instead of terribly. For instance, if you fear losing control and biting your partner's head off (literally), observe yourself handling the stress in a manner you can feel good about. When you finish your visualization (do it as long as it feels good—two minutes or twenty, it is up to you), affirm *aloud,* "My body knows how to have a baby. My labor and delivery unfold perfectly."

Make a list of everything you fear. Next to it, think of an action you can take to help ease that fear. For example:

FEAR	ACTION
Loss of control	Practice being less in control now
	Talk to partner about it being okay
Death of self or child	Reassure myself with statistics
	Think about how I could comfort myself if I did lose the baby
	Review my life and what I'm proud of
Episiotomy	Choose a health care provider who doesn't perform them on a regular basis
	Have my health care provider massage my perineum with warm oil compresses during birth
	Practice breathing so I can control pushing to ease my baby's head out
Hemorrhoids	Find out why they happen and how bad they are
	Buy cream and healing herbs
	Ask myself why I'm afraid

See Appendix: Herbs, Oils, and Other Natural Comforters.

Relax in a quiet place. Visualize your fear; whatever image or symbol spontaneously arises is perfect. It might not make logical sense. That's fine; you are looking for an emotional connection. See yourself placing this image or symbol in a box. Put the lid firmly on your fear. Then, visualize yourself decorating your box with images, objects, and things that make you feel supported, loved, and protected. As if you are creating a living decoupage. You might see a miniature version of your partner standing on the lid, smiling. You might envision the box being hugged by God, bathed in pearly light, or embellished with gold stars. Perhaps you see it adorned with all the knowledge about birth you have been gathering. Take your time; let your imagination go wild.

To finish, peek inside the box. See if the image of your fear has been altered or transformed. Perhaps it is smaller, less formidable, or has even disappeared. Don't be disappointed if the image is still potent. Just repeat this visualization again. The goal is not to deny or force your fear underground but to convince your conscious and unconscious mind that you are loved and supported, that you have resources.

The more you are able to confront your secret fears and anxieties, the better you will be prepared for the letting go of labor and the much bigger letting go of motherhood. Don't force yourself to let go. Don't avoid your darkest fears; don't rigidly keep everything together. Keep the idea "gently letting it open" in the back on your mind as you work with your fears. Stop when you are overwhelmed or panicked; push yourself when you feel you are not being honest with yourself.

Fear of Being a Terrible Mother

Unfortunately, the nasty fear of being a terrible mother tends to pop up for the rest of your life. However, during pregnancy and in the first few months after having the baby, it can be particularly debilitating.

During pregnancy, *get experience.* Visit a friend who is having a baby and help her. This is excellent training. Change diapers, doctor the umbilical cord, dress the baby, whatever seems particularly daunting. If you don't know anyone who is giving birth, extend your help to a woman in your childbirth education class (someone who is due several weeks or more before you) or see if there is an outreach program through a church, synagogue, or hospital in your area that might need volunteers to visit new moms. Note: If you do this and find the experience overwhelming or distasteful, don't put your baby up for adoption just yet. The element of motherly love, as ethereal as it always sounds, does change your attitude. The agony of someone else's puckered, wailing, sucking blob won't be nearly as overpowering when that prune is yours.

See Transforming Your Fears About Labor and Delivery; or Controlling Monkey Mind.

Ask yourself why you believe you will be a terrible mother. Because it sounds conceited and impossible to be a good one? Because of a trauma you experienced when you were young? Because you don't feel mature enough, smart enough, energetic enough, self-sacrificing enough? Because you don't have a job outside the home? Because you do have a job outside the home? Because you are too young? Or too old? Because you are alone? Because your relationship isn't perfect? Try a visualization around your fears. Do the fear-action list above or the meditation on placing your fear in a box.

Explore your relationship with your mother if you feel that is influencing your anxiety. (It does for many women.)

See I Want My Mommy.

The fear of being a horrible mother may come from trying to live up to a false image of perfection. "Women who try to submerge themselves into other people's notions of how they should mother, whether that other person is their husband, their mother, or an expert, will lose themselves and eventually their relationship with the child. Being good enough is what counts," writes Jane Price in *Motherhood: What It Does to Your Mind.* Start to define what being a good enough mother means to you by beginning to notice how you are already parenting your child. You are making decisions now regarding your needs and those of your child—whether to exercise or watch TV, eat chocolate or broccoli. You might say, "But see! I've already made mistakes. I can't be trusted." That is the point! You do make mistakes, you can't do everything perfectly, but still the baby survives and flourishes. But you say, "How do I know the baby is okay? How do I know I haven't already screwed up big-time?" All you can do is *trust yourself* and make a restless peace with this conundrum of parenting.

See What's Going to Happen to Me After the Baby Is Born?: The Myth of the Perfect Mother.

Get in the habit now, when you can find the energy, of quieting down and listening to your inner wisdom. This habit is an extraordinarily valuable mothering skill. Cultivate it now before the baby is born, or you will never find the time.

See The Spiritual Sustenance of Pregnancy: Strengthening Your Intuition.

Fears of being a terrible mother often stem from our beliefs that we aren't intrinsically good enough. Invest in your sense of self by caring for yourself as much as you can during this pregnancy.

Talk to other mothers of all ages. Ask them how they did an okay job. Ask them about their fears of being good enough. Visit a mother's group and listen.

See Nurturing Yourself During Pregnancy; How to Gracefully Ask for and Accept Support; Am I Fat and Ugly or Round and Beautiful?; and What's Going to Happen to Me After the Baby Is Born? for specific ideas.

Remember, you grow with the job. You don't know how to parent a toddler or a teenager when your child is born because you don't need to. You don't know how to parent two children before the second one is born because you haven't needed to. You will learn as the demand presents itself. Avoid making yourself anxious about not knowing what you don't need to know yet. "You dissolve your anxiety by doing this one day at a time," says Michele Wild, therapist and mother of three boys.

Fear of Losing Your Self

See What's Going to Happen to Me After the Baby Is Born?

Fear of losing my self was my biggest fear during pregnancy, and so I devoted a chapter to discussing it.

Resources:

A Child Is Born, by Linnart Nilsson (DTP, 1986). Extraordinary pictorial of life in utero.

Easier Childbirth, by Gayle Peterson (Shadow & Light Publications, 1999). Peterson is a pioneer in linking fear and problems during labor. This is the most accessible of her books and well worth checking out if fear still seems a mitigating issue.

Help, Comfort and Hope After Losing Your Baby in Pregnancy or the First Year, by Hannah Lothrop (Perseus, 1997). If through miscarriage, stillbirth, neonatal death, sudden infant death and termination of pregnancy, you lose your chid. Also for the caregivers who help through this heartbreak. The voices of other parents who have suffered the devastation of their baby's death are heard throughout this compassionate, insightful practical book.

The Places that Scare You: A Guide to Fearlessness in Difficult Times, by Pema Chodron (Shambhala, 2002). While this book has nothing to do with pregnancy, it is one of the best books for befriending fear.

Websites:

Pregnancy Dictionary
http://www.PregnancyDictionary.com

Consumer Reports Guide to Baby Products
http://www.consumerreports.org

Work

When to Do It:

- When you feel torn between staying home and your need to continue your work.

- If you are having trouble balancing work and pregnancy.

- If you always thought, "When I get pregnant, everything will fall into place, and I'll be able to balance work and motherhood," but now you are filled with panic, confusion, and perhaps anger at your mate for not struggling with the same conflict.

What Is It?

Working during pregnancy almost always gives a hint of what it is going to be like to work after you are a mom. Yes, negotiating for maternity leave and dealing with discrimination because of your pregnancy can be nasty, and the need to slow down and be good to ourselves can be almost impossible to arrange, but for most working women the real pressure comes from facing the looming question: "What will I do about work after the baby arrives?"

However, too many of us are stuck posing the question as "Should I work or not?" The real issue is, we deserve a full range of choices and support as working mothers. But most of us don't have this full range of options, and we don't necessarily believe we deserve them. We are left holding the bag: if we choose not to work, we question our self-worth, our value as role models, and may feel bored and cut off from "real life." If we continue to work (from necessity or

You'll Need:

Paper or pregnancy journal, and a pen.

Good books about being a working mom or a stay-at-home mom. See Resources.

Support from other women doing the same thing.

Excellent child care.

See What's Going to Happen to Me After the Baby Is Born? for more on identity and motherhood issues.

choice), we question whether we are damaging our children, we juggle phenomenal time pressures, and we rarely feel free from energy-draining guilt.

By trusting ourselves, our viewpoints, and our decisions and by working to have those decisions supported by our families and our society, we can decrease the conflict of being torn between mother-hood and self, motherhood and work. But where does this inner trust come from? From practice and from self-love. As namby-pamby as it may sound: if we love ourselves, we will trust ourselves, at least most of the time. Loving self-care fosters self-love and is especially critical during early motherhood. Doubting our choice to be a work-ing mother or a stay-at-home mother (and here is where the irony lies: we can't win either way) can cause us to question ourselves constantly, second-guess our ability to raise our child(ren), and make it difficult for us to see our children as independent people with separate emotional lives. We can end up perceiving everything they do as a direct result of our decision to work or not. That is too much pressure.

There is no way to know how you will feel about working until after the baby is here. But you need to lay the groundwork now to provide you with the maximum amount of options later. You need to start considering what work style would support you most as a mother. You need to think about how you can deal with the stressful pressure of being pulled in too many different directions. If staying home is an option, you must create regular breaks for yourself and an atmosphere of self-respect for the arduous job you are taking on. Being a wonder-ful mother means having a self to mother from. Giving this part of your life and identity some careful consideration during your preg-nancy can allow you to reap tremendous benefits later, even though you may be too ill or exhausted even to consider these issues right now or if you are absolutely sure you won't be working for ten years or you know you have no choice but to go right back to work because of that little nuisance called money.

Staying Afloat at Work While You're Pregnant

If you are working throughout most or all of your pregnancy, you may find yourself needing some extra help to cope. Try these tips:

Remember that taking care of yourself means you are taking care of your career. Think of yourself as an athlete in training. You have to be just as careful to eat well and at regular intervals and to get enough sleep and not exhaust yourself, or you won't be able to perform. This approach may mean cutting back a little on your time at work, taking one or two sick days. Remember that by cutting back a little, you are less likely to crash and need a huge rest. Guard your energy supply and concentration. You don't need to telegraph to your boss and co-workers that you are slowing down, but *you* must realize you now have different needs. Taking care of these needs will help you keep working.

A good office chair and some kind of footrest support are critical if you sit at your job for long hours. Get out of the habit of crossing your legs; it helps varicose veins develop. Stretch and take short walks around the office every hour for fatigue and to help prevent hemorrhoids. Do short amounts of work standing up, like returning phone calls. If you stand to do your job, investigate using a tall stool on wheels to give you a rest. Above all, get some excellent, supportive shoes.

If you are having a rough first trimester, consider taking some time off now to take care of yourself. You may feel you need to save that time for your maternity leave or for the end of your pregnancy, but for some women, a few days off in the early months is crucial for their sanity and job performance. Many women reported they wished they had taken time off in the beginning and then worked almost or right up to their due dates. "I spent the first three months dragging myself to the store and worried incessantly about keeping up. I took off three weeks before my due date, and after a week of preparing the nursery and getting birth announcements ready, I hated sitting around and waiting. I wish I had worked until the contractions started," noted Becka, mother of Jenna.

However, it is also possible to use your work as a way to keep from preparing mentally for labor and, more important, for the gigantic adjustment of becoming a mom. You must take enough time for yourself in the last two months, and especially the last month, to prepare psychologically. Try not to use work as a distraction from yourself.

If returning to work is currently your plan, start evaluating how supportive your boss and co-workers are and how flexible your working conditions are. Keep in mind: *flexibility is the most important asset for working parents*. Ask yourself:

- After I've announced my pregnancy, how is my boss treating me? How are my co-workers treating me? Do I feel supported or under siege?

- How easy is it for me to take time off to deal with the demands of pregnancy? (Examples could include mornings off for nausea, leaving early because of exhaustion, longer lunches for health care appointments.)

- How tied am I to being at work during strict office hours? How can I vary my routine? How easy is it to swap shifts or find someone to cover for me?

- Is there a regular morning meeting I must attend? (Mornings are when you will find yourself scrambling for an alternative sitter or dealing with a sick child.) Could it be rescheduled now (and couched in terms of everyone's convenience, not just yours)?

- What parts of my job are totally inflexible? Can I see myself being covered for those, in terms of child care, 95 percent of the time?

- Is there a big chunk of daily or weekly work that I do entirely on my own, without my boss needing me or without needing staff, files, or special equipment? Could I do this at home? Or could I arrange my work differently so that these chunks of independent work do exist?

- What skills can I acquire now, during my pregnancy, that would make my job more flexible and also make me more valuable to my employer? (Consider night courses, training seminars, and other avenues to expand your skills.)

Changing jobs or even careers during your pregnancy so that you will be more able to juggle life with baby sounds like as much fun as being thirteen again and having your mother cut your bangs. However, if your present job is completely lacking in flexibility, and your boss has made it clear he doesn't trust you to come back or to work as hard after the birth, you may want to consider this radical solution. Proceed slowly and keep in mind:

- Your sense of self-worth. You are entitled to a good job that supports you as a mother. Don't go job hunting with a low impression of yourself because you feel desperate. Pump yourself up: you are a brave, resourceful woman, and you have skills to offer. You are trying your best to fulfill your and your child's needs.

- Job searching is best done, for most women, during the middle of your pregnancy, when you often feel and look your best.

- Don't forget why you're putting yourself through this search. Your new job must offer what your old job doesn't: support for working moms. Don't forget to evaluate each opportunity on these grounds.

- If you work in a large company, consider a sideways move to a more flexible job.

- If you are taking the time to look for a job, you are obviously committed to returning to work. One way to stress this is to comment during interviews that you are an important (or sole) provider for your family.

- At interviews, people are legally forbidden to ask if you are married, how many children you have, and how many you plan to have.

- Tell everyone who interviews you that you are pregnant to avoid any miscommunication.

To Work or Not to Work: What Do You Really Want to Do?

> A working mother-to-be spends a lot of time justifying to herself her need to work. She wonders whether she really wants to be pregnant at all and dreams about rejecting the fetus. If she weren't pregnant, life could be so simple again. Because these fantasies of rejection are intolerable to her, they may take the form of fears about having damaged her baby.

So writes T. Berry Brazelton in *Working and Caring*. This may or may not be true for you. It was for me. I found that consciously exploring my options was the best strategy for examining the dilemma of motherhood versus work.

Find some quiet time when you have a little energy and are feeling perhaps a bit introspective. Arrange your writing materials nearby and relax with some deep breathing. Allow any tension to ebb out of your body and mind. Answer the questions below by letting everything you can think of flow out onto the page.

- Why do I work?

- Why do I work at the career/job that I do?

- How does my work make me feel? (Record your entire range of emotions.)

- In terms of work, if I could do anything, what would it be? (*No* restrictions.)

- If I could combine motherhood and working in an ideal way for me, without considering money, my partner's job, what my family or colleagues or friends would say, what would my life look like? What would a typical day consist of?

It may take several attempts to answer these tough questions. It may upset you. You may think, "I don't live in a perfect world, so stop teasing me by getting me to think about it." My goal is not to annoy or overwhelm you but to help you see beyond the obvious, beyond the strictures placed on you, and for you to let your dreams enter the picture.

What do you do with this knowledge? Discuss it with your partner. Meditate on what you've discovered. Pull together a brainstorming session with friends and people you respect in your community and other mothers faced with a similar predicament. Pose your problem and have everyone contribute possible solutions. Encourage all suggestions; nothing is too far-fetched. If you are staying home, find ways to fulfill your dreams and nourish your work self through making time for regular creative work, locating volunteer work that allows you to work directly with people and see the results of your efforts, and participating in professional associations and subscribing to professional journals. Work on believing mothers deserve more choices by taking political action to support what you want. Write a letter once a month to someone in legislative office. Work in your community to improve child care options. Join a political group that is striving for working mothers' rights.

Guilt and the Working Mother

If there is a working mother out there who doesn't feel conflicted and guilty on a regular basis, you must identify yourself as an endangered species. Seek protection quickly before the noxious, mucky, foul, vicious guilt monster eats you alive too. For the rest of us working moms, dealing with guilt (and time pressure) soon becomes an achingly awful part of life.

Here is a bit of solace to help you as you make decisions and plans, to soothe you if you already have a child or children and are working, or for down the road when you wake in middle of the night with a pounding heart, positive your baby is composing in her little mind her own version of *Mommy Dearest:*

The decision to go back to work is never final. You can always change your mind. Some women take three months off, work for three years, then take another year off. Or take a year off and work from then on. Or alternate periods of intense career focus with their husbands or partners, so that someone is available to parent three-quarters of the time. There are endless combinations of working and full-time mothering. Nothing is written in stone.

Whatever your reasons for working, *if they are important to you*, they are valid.

You are not alone. About 59 percent of women return to work outside the home after their child is born.

When it is time to go back to work, whether after six weeks or six years, locate other mothers who have gone through and are going through this same, often painful, transition. Talking about how your child regressed back to crawling upon being left at day care or your jealousy of your child's relationship with the baby-sitter helps you see these events for what they are: *normal*. Share your diminishing feelings of competency, the feeling that the day care personnel or grandma or the housekeeper knows better, and, of course, your worry, your guilt. Isolation is your enemy.

It might comfort you to know that no matter what you do, someone is going to frown on you. That is the bane of being a mother. If you stay home, former colleagues and friends might say, "What do you *do* all day long?" judging you inferior to a working woman. If you work, someone is going to conclude you are a shoddy, selfish mother (and it is obviously none of their business). Get it straight from the start that you will not please everyone, including perhaps your immediate family. To try to please everyone will only cause you heartache.

Mothers who achieve balance shun perfection. *Reasonable* expectations is the most vital phrase to imprint on your brain. It isn't that you can't "have it all" (although I've never been sure exactly what that meant); you just can't "have it all" perfectly and done by only you right this minute. Realistic expectations, an equal partner, if you have one, a good support system including good child care, a sense that your work is fulfilling to you, and regular self-nurturing make up a workable recipe.

Support Is Crucial

Working mothers have less stress if they are supported by their partners (and single working mothers by their chosen support team), if they have child care they feel good about, and if their workplace is supportive and flexible. Now, during your pregnancy, is the time to strengthen each of these areas. Read about being a working parent. Start looking for child care *early*. Do not assume it will be easy. Even more than having a flexible job, having excellent, reliable child care is what will make the difference in your working life. Finding good child care it is a giant subject, so I've left it to the experts.

See Resources.

The best advice I've encountered on child care is to consider not how you can replace yourself but how you can *complement* yourself. "A caregiver can be good enough when he or she is not expected to be ideal in all capacities but simply in those where the parent needs help most," writes Melinda Marshall in *Good Enough Mothers*. Marshall suggests we consider some hard questions when looking for child care: what we are unable to give our children and what we want to give our children. No parent readily wants to admit weakness or, even more horrible, what we are unwilling to give or sacrifice. But by not confronting our own weaknesses and desires we will never be happy with the child care we do find because we have unrealistic expectations for ourselves and impose these on our day care. What if, when setting out to find child care, you considered what your children must have that you are not in position to provide? Don't let what's available curtail your imagination and active choice. Instead, consider what kind of child care would benefit your child the most, what kind of child care would fill in where you cannot, and then mesh that with the demands of your work. It's not easy, but it helps to think through all of your options and make conscious choices.

Constantly remind yourself that balancing work and children is not a question for moms, it is a question for *parents*. We automatically assume Mom will have to make career sacrifices and changes, not Dad. Changing this fundamental mindset, both within ourselves and within our society, is perhaps the most important step we can take. This work is linked to self-care in pregnancy because as we come to believe we are worthwhile, wonderful creatures, we realize we are entitled to equal treatment as mothers.

See Nurturing Yourself During Pregnancy; Tumultuous, Turbulent Feelings; How to Gracefully Ask for and Accept Support; Am I Fat and Ugly or Round and Beautiful?; Forming Your Support Team; The Spiritual Sustenance of Pregnancy; and What's Going to Happen to Me After the Baby Is Born? for ways to strengthen your belief that you deserve equal choices.

Talk as openly as you can with your partner about your beliefs and family influences concerning raising children, working mothers, and

See Connecting with Your Partner: Expectations for help having these discussions.

father's involvement. Get down to what each of you believes is right, good, wholesome. If you must work, it is not uncommon for a man to feel threatened that he can't provide the entire family income and for you to feel angry that you must work. These emotions don't make you a throwback to Tupperware parties, but they must be discussed. Talk about how you were each raised, what you think is normal. Whether you were brought up in an city apartment or a suburban house or a sprawling farm, with a working mom or a stay-at-home mom or an absent father—these are all going to influence deeply your ideas about women working. It is not uncommon for very old-fashioned ideas about what a mother is to push into your lives—from both of your psyches. The danger is leaving these feelings unsaid and waiting for them to strike after the baby is born.

Negotiating Your Maternity Leave

Under the Pregnancy Discrimination Act of 1978, it is illegal to fire or refuse to hire you because you are pregnant, and if you are working you are entitled to paid disability. An employer cannot make you use your vacation time before your leave benefits take effect, nor can he or she treat your benefits differently if you are single mom. Under The Family and Medical Leave Act of 1993, if you work for a company with more than fifty employees, you are guaranteed an unpaid pregnancy or adoption leave of twelve weeks, and your job must be held for your return. That's the law, but there are plenty of loopholes. According to a 1994 survey by the Families and Work Institute, only 16 percent of women found their supervisors supportive, and only 7 percent of women found their co-workers supportive of the need to take off time for family!

Before you tell *anyone* at work you are pregnant, do some detective work. Is there a set policy for maternity leave? How many weeks paid? If your company is small, how many, if any, weeks unpaid while your job is still guaranteed? Don't automatically assume you are lucky to get any leave. If necessary, work on your sense of entitlement, balanced by what you believe is fair and possible for your company. As subtly as possible, find out what has happened to other pregnant women and mothers. If you hear one horror story after another, now might be the time to consider looking for a new job (see page 161 for ideas on how to do that when pregnant). If no one at your level of employment has been pregnant, like it or not, you're going to be a trailblazer.

Before you approach your boss to talk about maternity leave, be prepared with specific ideas for your situation. Consider your leave from your employer's perspective. Put yourself in your company's shoes. For example, if your company offers six weeks at full pay, but you want to take off four months, perhaps you can offer to do work at home, to work part-time, to job-share with another new mother, or to find a temporary replacement worker. Dream up creative solutions and remember, if you don't ask, you'll never know. You can't be positive how you will feel about working after the baby is born; six weeks can sound like an eternity B.B. (before baby) and feel like an afternoon once your leave is almost over. Waiting as long as possible to reveal your pregnancy and using that time to do some research (reading and talking to other working moms) as well as thinking about what your minimum requirements and maximum desires are puts you in a better bargaining position. What you *don't* want to do is negotiate the least amount of time and then find out you need more. Offering reasonable ideas to solve the problem (I hate to label pregnancy as a problem, but that is the way most businesses perceive it) before your company even knows it has one might thwart a Grinch that wants to steal your job.

From the first breaking of your news, keep your radar finely tuned to pick up everyone's reactions, and add that information to your findings. In a larger, more formal work situation, you might need to schedule an appointment to discuss specifics after giving your boss the news. Come prepared with your own proposals for your return to work. Outline your ideas, but also don't be afraid to ask questions as well, like how your boss sees your maternity leave affecting your career and your chances for promotion, if he or she feels you won't be able to continue at the same pace or on the same assignment when you return, and who will cover your work while you are gone. When you've agreed on your leave, confirm the plan in a memo.

Near the end of your pregnancy, discuss reentry with your boss and co-workers. Will a transition period be rough for anyone? Reassure them that you will do your part. Reinforce that you will be returning. Make remarks like, "When I return from leave, that will be about the time we'll be writing the new catalog copy" or "I'm looking forward to working on that project in the spring" or "I don't think it will take me long to get up to speed on the new computer program."

During your leave, keep in touch. Have lunch with co-workers and catch up on gossip. Visit work before and after your lunch. Keep the conversation minimally on your new baby. On the other hand, be careful to protect your leave and this extraordinary time with your newborn. Keep your visits primarily social. It is too easy to be sucked into taking care of the office by taking work home. Unless it is absolutely vital to your long-term career, don't work until your leave is over. Delight in this unstructured time with your baby. Nap.

Guilt and the Stay-at-Home Mom

Society gives us a choice as women that it still doesn't fully grant men: the ability to stop working and stay at home with our children, if we can support ourselves or someone can support us. For most stay-at-home moms, the internal struggle is one of validation: am I still worthwhile even though I don't work or don't have a professional identity? Other struggles include justifying the time you take off for yourself, dealing with isolation, and receiving less support from partners because everything to do with the house and child(ren) can quickly become "your" territory.

See Preparing for Postpartum for specific ways to plan down time.

Meeting other moms and forming a baby-sitting co-op can help eliminate isolation and the anxiety of having no time off. Besides slavery or indentured servitude, there are no other jobs in the world that offer as little free time as mothering. But to be an effective mom, you must, must, *must* have time to recharge! Believe this if you believe nothing else in this book. Make concrete plans for how you will acquire alone time in your postbaby life. "The pervasive myth of the self-sacrificing mother, coupled with the very real demands placed on caretakers by young children and the repetition of work in the home, can undermine a woman's confidence in a life of her own and her sense of personal accomplishment," notes Darcie Sanders and Martha Bullen in *Staying Home*. In other words, it is remarkably easy to find yourself with the self-esteem of a cockroach. The need to keep a little space and time for yourself is critical for all moms, but especially ones new to the role.

Be as clear as you can about your reasons for staying home. Be as clear as possible that your baby is not your career. Your self-worth cannot reside in your child. Your desire to be a great mom and do the best for your baby can slowly and insidiously become a way to show that you still have worth. How soon your baby rolls over, sits up, walks, even teethes, eats solids, or what she wears, can all feel like signs of whether you are doing your job well enough, ways to prove you are a worthwhile person. You must create outside reinforcement for the part of you that is not a mom.

Forget guilt. I know it's ridiculously easy to say and incredibly hard to do. Consider Diane's comment, mother of two: "Darwin is five and a half, and that is old enough to see how his personality is. He's a great kid. It has taken that long to see that I did a good job, that staying home has been worth it." Another woman commented, "Some days I do a good job, some days I don't. Some days I love it, some days I hate it." Obliterate those expectations that to be a good mom, you are supposed to love every minute of it. No one does. I repeat, no one does.

Explore what you believe about being a good mother. This is extremely important because the myth of being a perfect mom can descend and smother us.

See What's Going to Happen to Me After the Baby Is Born?: The Myth of the Perfect Mother.

If you have worked before, a sometimes difficult issue to deal with is how you and your partner will emotionally and financially handle your not bringing in an income. Money is power, and for many women, not controlling their own income or not contributing to the family pot can cause waves of guilt and put new pressure on the relationship. Few couples are willing to explore this quagmire, but it is essential to set aside time to look at it, for the guilt often doesn't set in right away. Suddenly, after you haven't been working for a few months, a conflict may erupt over a major purchase or over money for a movie. One solution is for mom to be paid a "salary" that goes into an account (or envelope) of her own. This is money to be spent on mom and mom alone, without having to ask anyone or feel guilty.

Resources:

Flux: Women on Sex, Work, Love, Kids, and Life in a Half-Changed World, by Peggy Orenstein and Alice Van Straalen (Knopf, 2001). Interviews with hundreds of women about how they combine work and family; how they navigate society and personal perceptions of what women should do.

Life's Work: Confessions of an Unbalanced Mom, by Lisa Belkin (Touchstone Books, 2003). Witty personal essays about the collision between work and kids.

Nursing Mother, Working Mother: The Essential Guide for Breastfeeding and Staying Close to Your Baby After You Return to Work, by Gale Pryor (Harvard Common Press, 1997). Very helpful advice on how to continue breastfeeding.

Reinventing Ourselves After Motherhood: How Former Career Women Refocus Their Personal and Professional, by Susan Lewis (McGraw-Hill, 2000). Light hearted, realistic, like talking to a wise friend.

Staying Home, by Darcie Sanders and Martha M. Bullen (Spencer & Waters, 2001). Offers help in making the transition from working professional to full-time mom. How to set up a baby-sitting co-op.

Staying Home Instead, by Christine Davidson (Jossey-Bass, 1998). Guidelines for how to become a one-paycheck household.

The Working Mother's Guide to Life: Strategies, Secrets, and Solutions, by Linda Mason (Three Rivers Press, 2002). All encompassing manual with a slant toward middle-class mothers with partners.

Websites:

Blue Suit Mom
http://www.bluesuitmom.com

Working Moms Refuge
http://www.momsrefuge.com

The New Homemaker
http://www.thenewhomemaker.com

Moms Helping Moms
http://www.MomsHelpMoms.com

Home Based Working Moms
http://www.hbwm.com

Mom's Network— A work-at-home mom's community
www.momsnetwork.com

I Want My Mommy

Reaching Out and Mothering Yourself

When to Do It:

- If you feel vaguely lonely or sad and want to reach out to your mom, but when you do it doesn't quite satiate you.

- When you wish to learn about and join the lineage of mothers that begot you.

- When you want to curl up on the couch with your blankie and never get up.

- If your mother is deceased.

What Is It?

"When I found out I was pregnant, I experienced a real crisis. It came to me I needed to spend time with my mother. I really needed to be taken care of. I went home and was able to be egoless with my mother for the first time. I finally got what I needed, which was to be cherished as a little girl." Wendy's story relates the poignant, urgent need many pregnant women and new moms feel: the need to be mothered. To lie on the couch and be fed Jell-O. To cuddle close and listen to the thunder, knowing that nothing can hurt you. To let go of the need to be in control, to be right, to plan every moment of your life, because someone else will take care of it for you. To be dependent without worrying whether you will be hurt or changed by the experience. To feel utterly safe, contented, fulfilled. This is the longing for mommy love.

You'll Need:

Your journal or paper, and a pen.

"For a mother to respond to her infant's complete dependence on her, she must reexperience and work through the longing she once had toward her own mother," writes Jane Swigart in *The Myth of the Bad Mother*. Having a baby can conjure up the desire to experience an ever-lasting, all-giving font of unconditional love and the rage of being thwarted in that desire. We want to be loved and nurtured, to relive that cuddly, warm, perfect security. Giving birth can also bring to light aspects of your relationship with your mother and memories of how you were mothered. If your mother is dead or you have a particularly bruising relationship with her, pregnancy and motherhood can make your wounds feel fresh and newly distressing.

The longing for mother love is activated with a vengeance anywhere from the second trimester to (and especially) the fourth trimester—your first months postpartum. Poignant questions arise: "Who is going to look after me?" "Do I have to grow up?" "Am I still special?" This yearning is the wake-up call to mother yourself—to understand how desperately each human being wants to be loved, held, and protected and to create that love for yourself. Mothering yourself may include making peace with your mother and seeing her as an individual. Perhaps more important, mothering ourselves is digesting the possibility that the yearning for mother love may, at its heart, be about the elusive search for spiritual connection, the soul of self-nurturing.

What to Do:

What Do You Want from a Mother?

The first step in mothering ourselves is to discover what we want from a mother. I say "a" mother to remind us that there are many levels to being mothered, not all of them having to do with our real-life moms.

The questions below are for contemplation. When you feel the desire to be mothered or to reach out to your mother, stop and cogitate on the first question. Relax and let it develop in your mind. If you find your mind wandering (which is normal), return to the issue at hand by gently focusing on the question again.

- What do I yearn for a mother to give me right now?

If an action or need occurs to you, then ask yourself:

- Can my real mother give this to me, or is it more appropriate (or only possible) to ask someone else? Or can I give this to myself? If none of these is possible, is there a way I can make peace with not having this yearning fulfilled?

For example, in her sixth month of pregnancy, Shawn found herself dreaming about her mother almost every night. "I wanted to call her every day, which is unusual for me. I felt this compulsion to be with mommy, but I wasn't sure what I wanted from her." Shawn contemplated the question "What do I yearn for a mother to give me right now?" and two things popped into her head: permission to nap without feeling guilty and permission to quit work. "I was shocked. I am very committed to my career and to working after the baby is born." Shawn explored her findings further using the additional questions. "The word *permission* kept leaping out at me. I saw how much I was still waiting for my mom to validate my life, to tell me I was doing good. I realized I was going to have to start doing that for myself, and quick. Work was harder to figure out, but after contemplating this subject in my journal over several weeks, I saw I wanted to feel I *could* quit, that someone would take care of me and the baby. That was so hard for me to own up to—I'm very independent. I knew intellectually that I could not quit, and most of me didn't want to, yet I needed to discuss with my partner this need to feel taken care of. We decided I should try to take a longer maternity leave, that he would bring me breakfast in bed on the weekends and go to my prenatal appointments with me. We also started looking more carefully at our finances."

Bobbie is a single mother who has a difficult relationship with her mother. She found herself feeling depressed and cranky toward the end of her pregnancy. She meditated on the question over several walks in the woods. "It was very hard for me to even consider needing anything from my mother, so asking myself what I yearned for from 'a' mother helped. Still, it took a while before anything came to me. Dimly but insistently, it kept coming into my mind that I needed to talk to my mother about her childhood. I had absolutely no intention of doing that. So I didn't. I had Robyn and everything was fine, until

See Postbirth Nourishment: Surviving the Emotions.

about three weeks postpartum, when I got very sad and lonely. I suddenly resented Robyn's demands and just wanted to be taken care of myself. I'm so lucky I had my best friend around. Nancy visited every day after work, brought meals, got me to take baths, while she watched the baby. She also talked me into seeing a therapist. Turns out, part of my therapy homework was to interview my mom about her childhood. I found out things I had never known before, things that made me realize why she had always been so cold and distant. There wasn't any fairy-tale ending. My point is I wish I had talked to her when I was pregnant. I wish I had given more thought to how I needed to be mothered before Robyn arrived."

Explore your yearnings as many times as it feels appropriate. Don't force yourself to do anything you don't feel ready to do. But if you want to act on your ideas yet need help, *please* ask a friend or professional. Little attention has been paid to the tremendous strain of becoming a mother, but one thing is certain: the mother needs to be mothered, whether by her biological mother or a friend, if she is to mother her infant.

Postpartum

Ask yourself again:

• What do I yearn for a mother to give me right now?

If an action or need occurs to you, then ask yourself:

• Can my real mother give this to me, or is it more appropriate (or only possible) to ask someone else? Or can I give this to myself? If none of these is possible, is there a way I can make peace with not having this yearning fulfilled?

Be especially sensitive and sweet with yourself. You are going through enormous changes, some of which you might not digest for years. The need to be mothered is strongest now, perhaps the strongest it has been since you were an infant. Give yourself what you need! You don't have to do it alone. Please don't tough it out.

If your mother is deceased, you can experience the sorrow of her death anew with the birth of your child, especially if this is your first. Or you may find yourself depressed when your child reaches the age you were when your mother died. Being conscious of this possibility and allowing yourself to grieve again can help prevent a lingering or debilitating depression from setting in.

What Was It Like for Your Mother as a Mother?

Understanding your mother's experience of mothering can offer great insight into your own expectations about how you will mother.

Engage your mother over photos of you as an infant. Ask your mom,

• How did becoming a mom change you?

See if certain photos suggest specific questions. For example, a photo of your mom, your grandmother, and you as a infant might prompt you to ask, "Did Grandmother help you after I was born?"

If you have an older sibling, you might want to ask the same question over photos of him or her. If your mother is dead or your relationship is too strained, find another source to talk with, perhaps your grand-mother, aunt, cousin, or a friend of your mother's.

You might also want to ask:

• What did you want from your mother when you were pregnant and when you were a new mom?

• What did you want from your mother that she couldn't give you? (If you are aware that your mother did not or does not have a good relationship with her mother.)

• What was it like for you to be a mother?

• In what ways did you try to raise me differently than your mother raised you? How did you set out to do it differently?

• What do you still wish your mother could give to you?"

These questions can be enlightening when asked of your mother alone, and they are powerful when posed to your mother, grandmother, and perhaps an aunt at the same time.

Forgiving Our Mothers for Being Less than Perfect

Our vision of motherhood is largely shaped by the way we were mothered, which of course means imperfectly. But *of course* implies we accept the imperfection of our mothers. Most of us, if we could admit to it, don't. We wish we had been mothered perfectly. We may feel a little miffed about it, if not downright angry. Judith Schwartz sums up our complex relationship with our mothers and the need for perfection brilliantly in *The Mother Puzzle:*

> We began our lives in a perfectly solipsistic state: the world revolved around us, it *existed* for us, particularly our mothers, who were the part of the world that we knew best. Therefore, we've needed to accept three myths: the idea of maternal self-sacrifice (when young, we *expected* those sacrifices; later on, we wanted to believe they were appropriate so we won't feel guilty for having forced them upon our mothers); the belief in an innate, unvarying maternal instinct (wasn't our mothers' purpose in life to give birth to and care for us?); and the notion of maternal fulfillment (isn't creating *us* enough for one mortal human to achieve in life?). Similarly, we've needed to see mother as all-good and all-knowing (if she's not, who is?) and asexual (any sexual needs would detract from *our* specialness in life).

Ask yourself if any of these three myths are true for you. Did you believe or do you still believe your mother's true purpose in life is or was to be there for you? The answer may well be no. Great, you are that much further along in seeing your mother as a mortal. For me, the answer was, deep down, shamefully, yes. I still believed my mom's true purpose in life was to take care of me, especially when I was sick. When I compared the thesis of this book—that total self-sacrifice is not necessary to be a good mother, to what I believed, I began to see my double standard: the sacrifices my mother had made for me were

part of her job description but *not* part of mine. In my thirties and a
mother myself, I still considered my mother more of an icon, an eter-
nal comforter, than a person.

Here are a few active steps to take in forging a more accurate and forgiving perception of your mother.

Note: If you have had an abusive or extraordinarily painful relationship with your mother, or if your mother has died, please proceed
with care.

Contemplate the question: In what ways do I want to mother differently than my mother?

Then, choose one issue that comes up, the one you feel most strongly
about. As an example, imagine your list includes not being overprotective and fearful.

Free-associate for ten minutes in your journal about how your mother
was overprotective of you. Write about your disappointments, about
what you want to do differently and why.

Put this away for a few days. Reread it while putting yourself in your
mom's shoes. Ask yourself:

How did the era in which my mother lived make her overprotective
and fearful? Consider the historical and cultural influences, anything
from World War II and the atomic bomb to tight sweaters and
romance novels, to rampant drugs and rock 'n' roll.

What choices in life did my mom have, especially financially? How
did her range of choices (or lack of choices) shape her when it came to
being overprotective or fearful?

How did her relationship with my father (biological, adopted, or
stepfather, whoever is most important by presence or absence) influence her?

What positive things did I get from being overprotected?

How did the way my grandmother raised her affect her on this issue?

Some patterns will be very obvious, others less so. Spend a few minutes trying to see things through your mother's eyes. See where that leads you.

Consider how you have idealized your mother. Turn your image of your mother over in your mind. Think about her before you go to bed and see what your dreams reveal. Jump-start your memory by looking at childhood photos, visiting childhood haunts, hugging old toys. When you get a good picture of your idealization, consider how it serves you as a mother, and how it serves your relationship with your mother. Does it put too much pressure on you to live up to this ideal? If so, what specific parts of the ideal can you let go of? Does it make it hard to relax around your mother? On the positive side, does your idealization create a rosy role model? Consider what qualities you wish to replicate as a mother. Finally, ask yourself how our culture has shaped your picture of your mother.

See Resources for books on forgiving your mom.

What disappointments in your life do you feel your mother is responsible for? Are you willing to make a list? The best way to do this is to sit down and very quickly write down everything that comes to mind. Shock yourself with all the things, big and petty, you are willing to blame your mom for. Next, study your list. Can you link your expectations of yourself as a mother, of your own maternal responsibility, to these disappointments your mother may or may not have caused? It may not be clear at first; you may have to let it percolate for a bit. Pinpoint how much control, input, and knowledge your mother really had over your life. How much is she *really* to blame? When you stop believing she is all-knowing and all-powerful, you have to start seeing how much of your life you are responsible for and how other people affected you, and perhaps how little your mother could actually do. Finally (and you might not be able to do this easily or until several months postbaby), forgive your mother for every disappointment you can honestly hold her responsible for.

How has the ideal of a perfect mother tyrannized or wounded your mother? How has her own quest for perfection, her own inability to accept her mistakes, driven her? What do you wish you could tell her to help her relax and accept herself? Say it out loud. Can you follow your own advice?

Your mother also experienced the postpartum wilderness. Can you imagine what it was like for her? Does that help you understand her and her relationship with you? Find out what it was like directly after your birth from whomever you can ask.

Mother Yourself

Meditate on the self-mothering ideas gathered here. Some are more poetic than practical; others may offend your independent nature. Let them enliven your very personal search to find ways to meet the difficult-to-name, shadowy, slippery longing to be mothered.

What aspects of your own childhood do you wish to try to give to your coming baby? In addition to the practical (safe home, college education), pay attention to the emotional (self-esteem, courage) and the very personal (a Pooh Bear, classical music playing at Christmas). Give yourself a taste of these things now.

Locate a protected place in nature to rest—a hollow tree high on a hill, a shallow, sun-warmed tide pool at the ocean's edge, a cave in the earth. Lie there. Listen for the heartbeat of the Earth. Let yourself be an infant of the Great Mother.

Dig a hole in the Earth (a sandy beach is wonderful) and lay your belly in it. Let the Earth cradle you.

Give yourself a security object. It could be an organic cotton blanket, a lucky marble you carry in your pocket, a special scent that makes you feel protected and caressed.

Ask a loved one to say no to that volunteer job you don't want to do, to turn away the teenager selling magazine subscriptions, to run interference between you and the world for a day or two.

Ask someone else to celebrate your womanly body. Have someone brush your hair for a very long time. Or give you a scalp massage. Or paint your toenails. Or pat your back while you are going to sleep. Open up and take it in!

Find someone you trust to listen to you and occasionally mirror back important points but otherwise to listen without interrupting or adding his or her two cents. Agree to a specified period of time. Drink in the attention.

Create a bedtime ritual that makes you feel loved. Reciting a childhood prayer, sleeping with a stuffed animal, and wearing well-worn flannel pj's are possibilities.

Getting Practical Help from Your Mother Postpartum

Many women ask their mothers to come be with them or help with baby-sitting at the emotionally raw and exciting time of postpartum. You may find yourself needing your mother's wisdom and reassurance at this time like never before. However, a bit of preparation can avert disaster.

Start deciding how you envision your mother (sister, aunt, best friend) helping you. Project yourself past the birth of your child. Do you see her taking care of the house and food, leaving you to be alone with your new baby? Do you see her teaching you how to care for the little creature?

What are your expectations? How do you envision relating to your mother? Watch out if you are expecting a magical transformation of your relationship with your mother. Sore spots, age-old feuds, and rancorous disappointments do not disappear overnight because of a birth. It is a miracle and it will mold your relationship into a new shape, but often in slow, subtle ways. Be very clear what your expectations are and make sure they are *very* realistic.

When do you see her coming? The day after the birth? A week before? Two weeks after? For women with partners, the hard part hits when he or she goes back to work. For moms who have a C-section, help is needed immediately. For veteran moms, immediate help with older siblings is often most important. If this is your first baby, you can't be sure when your mom's help will be most useful. Talk to a few friends. Ask them what they did or wish they would have done differently. Many women report they wanted someone to take care of them, especially in the first few weeks, so they could focus on the baby. If a colicky or fussy period started or when sleep deprivation built up, starting from two to six weeks, then they wanted spells away from baby.

How long do you see her staying? Again, watch your expectations. If you have always gotten into a humdinger of a fight after three days, and yet you are expecting two blissful weeks, maybe you need to build in a breather.

Where do you imagine her staying? Again, most women assume in their own home is the only answer, but think about your privacy needs, if necessary your mom's (aunt's, sister's, best friend's) relationship with your partner, and how much space you have. One woman rented a single apartment across the street from her house for a month so her mother could be by herself for a few hours each evening. Sally's mother signed up with a vacation house–swapping service, swapping her house for a month with a house near Sally. Ellen's friend spent most of her time at her boyfriend's house, so Ellen borrowed her friend's apartment for her mother to get away to from time to time and get a full night's sleep.

Once you have given this matter ten or fifteen minutes of thought and perhaps discussed it with your partner or a friend, communicate what you wish to your mother in the most loving and nonjudgmental way you can. Pick a time when nobody is tired or angry about something else. It is a good idea to discuss arrangements early in your pregnancy so that your mother doesn't form expectations that might conflict with your plans. Do keep in mind your mother's (aunt's, sister's, best friend's) needs. Try to put yourself in her shoes.

See Forming Your Support Team: Getting Support from Your Family.

Resources:

Living A Connected Life: Creating and Maintaining Relationships that Last a Lifetime, by Kathleen A. Brehony (Owl Books, 2003). A well-written and well-researched guide for creating and deepening the vital relationships that give life richness and meaning.

Motherless Daughters, by H. Edelman (Delta, 1995). If your mother is deceased, read this book.

The Common Thread: Mothers, Daughters, and the Power of Empathy, by Martha Manning (William Morrow, 2002). A thoughtful, beautifully written exploration of the many "squares" in the quilt of mother daughter relationships.

The Feminine Face of God: The Unfolding of the Sacred in Women, by Patricia Hopkins and Sherry Ruth Anderson (Bantam, 1992). Exquiste soul food.

The Poetic Side
of Pregnancy

Creativity, Dreams, and the Need for Beauty

When to Do It :

- When you feel dull, frumpy, or boring.

- When you are experiencing intense nighttime or daytime dreams.

- If you feel full of magic and mystery: visions, oracles, inventions.

What Is It ?

To be pregnant is to be immersed in a profoundly creative state, a transformation that cries out to be celebrated. Some women find themselves feeling extraordinarily creative. Most women find their dreams are much more vivid and easier to recall, providing all kinds of tantalizing clues to their feelings and fears about becoming a mother. Many women interviewed talked about the need to nest, to create a beautiful environment in their homes, or to be around beauty, to "soak up museums, galleries, music, movies, even shop windows," as one woman put it. Jean Shinoda Bolen writes in her autobiography, *Crossing to Avalon,* "Pregnancy is like the creativity that comes from making a descent into one's own depth, in which the person is changed in the process of bringing forth the work—creative work that comes out of the soul and is the child of it. This experience of pregnancy and this process of creativity can be symbolized by the labyrinth found near the entrances to ritual caves and on the floors of cathedrals, which are

You'll Need :

Pregnancy or dream journal, and pen.

Drawing paper and butcher paper large enough to lie on with room to spare around you.

Art materials like paints, markers, crayons, old jewelry, leaves, found objects, photos, pieces of cloth.

womb-like spaces." You may want to give expression to the dreams and feelings springing from the visionary place where you stand.

But life can be remarkably busy, especially if you are preparing for the second child, arranging details for the birth, and getting caught up with work. All of this takes energy, perhaps leaving you with little energy for tending to your creative urges and feeding your aesthetic hunger. This chapter is intended not to make you feel you must do something, but to give you direction if you feel creative.

What to Do:

Shaping a Resplendent World—Nesting

Anna Bunting, a midwife living in Santa Barbara, has a vision of a divine place where pregnant women go to relax, "especially toward the end of your pregnancy." You cross an ornate bridge over a cool stream and enter a glorious, tranquil oasis where everything is beautiful. You are wrapped in soft, multicolored robes; outdoor pavilions have fluttering white curtains, you enjoy music playing, sunshine, hummingbirds, orange blossoms blooming. . . . Everything exists to pamper and soothe you.

Look around your life and see how you can create your own version of Anna's place. You may come up with recovering an old chair, driving a different route to work, lining your drawers with scented paper, framing a favorite prayer or affirmation to hang over the kitchen sink, starting a book of memorable quotes about being a mother, studying the night sky, getting your shoes polished and dyed, taking a painting class at your local museum, buying a flowering houseplant, throwing out half your furniture and living like a monk, lighting scented candles every night for a few minutes before bed, organizing your photos in an album, or reading Annie Dillard while lying in a hammock by the ocean. I had such a need for fresh flowers that I became obsessed with going to the farmer's market every Saturday to buy them. One of my pregnancy rituals was arranging them every few days, changing their water, moving them around the house. Sometimes I felt I was possessed by Martha Stewart, but I let myself enjoy this flower fetish all the same.

Don't dismiss your aesthetic needs or your nesting urges. Like your enhanced emotions, these are a product not just of hormones, but of legitimate needs. However, you must understand that your mate, your best friend, and your mother do not feel the intensity that you do to find the perfect set of 250-thread-count sunflower-patterned sheets or to stroll the botanical garden every day at twilight. You can ask others to support you, but you cannot ask them to share your passion.

Call a "nesting meeting" with your family members. Explain to them what you would like them to do to help you with your need for more beauty, order, or cleanliness. For younger children, relate your desire to something they have wanted very badly. When space or taste differences are causing conflict, ask for the compromise of designating one room, corner, or wall as yours to do with as you please.

See The Spiritual
Sustenance of Pregnancy:
Establish a Reminder.

Taking on big environment-improving projects can be risky. Be careful that your desire for beauty and order isn't mutating into stifling perfectionism. Having the baby's room painted is important, but having someone paint the outside of the house may be less important than spending time relaxing with your mate. (Pregnant women should not be exposed to paint fumes.) Having lovely baby furniture may seem crucial, but the money saved by accepting hand-me-downs might reduce your stress more.

Many women find themselves needing to move. This can be stressful enough (we moved ninety-five miles north to a new town when I was six months pregnant), but unless you absolutely *must* add a room or otherwise do a major remodeling job, unless you are *sure* you have enough money, and unless you have *no* choice, avoid remodeling or building a new house while you are pregnant. It is a sublime torture known only to modern Superwomen. In addition, the chemicals used during remodeling can be dangerous to your unborn child.

Look to Your Dreams

Research done on dreaming during pregnancy has shown pregnant women dream more vividly, remember their dreams more easily, and also seem to have dreams that offer more tangible and accessible insights. Your dreams may chart your acceptance of the baby, the growing reality of the awesome change that is rapidly approaching. They can allow you to acknowledge hidden fears and problems, giving you clues to what work you need to do in life to prepare. Dreams offer potent symbols, spiritual growth, and comfort, if you wish to explore them.

Dreams during pregnancy demand to be recorded. They seem too precious to forget (I write this although I have always had great resistance to writing down and working with my dreams). In a special notebook or in your pregnancy journal, jot down your dreams every morning, starting *tomorrow*. The habit is important. Write the dream in the present tense, as if it were again unfolding around you. Even brief scraps are useful.

When you have a small supply of recorded dreams, make a list of recurring objects, people, or events by browsing quickly through the dreams. Study the list for a motif. What thread or threads run through your dreams? What does this pattern want to tell you? Write a poem using the elements on this list. Don't worry about using the dreams in the order you dreamed them. Let your mind wander and make new connections. Read the poem several days later and ask yourself, "What can I learn about my pregnancy (or labor, birth, or baby) from this poem?"

Draw, paint, or make a collage of a dream or part of a dream to explore a specific concern you have. Choose a dream that has a lot of energy for you, a dream that has stayed with you. Ask yourself, "What images or elements stand out most in my mind? What is the most vivid part of the dream? What is the central emotion?" Gather your art materials (whatever you have, whatever you can afford, whatever appeals to you), and, keeping in mind the images and emotions of your dream, create a dream landscape. Use the image as a meditation point. See what feelings or thoughts occur to you as you live with this image.

An alternative: share dreams with your mate. Take your mate's dream and do this art exploration with his or her dream. You can also do this with a friend or relative who is pregnant. Finally, you could do it with your mother or a significant woman in your life who remembers a dream from her pregnancy. Share your images afterward and discuss your interpretations.

Have a dream interview with your mate, close friend, or sister who shares an interest in your pregnancy. Describe your dream in the present tense. Don't leave anything out, but also try not to embellish. Your dream interviewer listens carefully. Then your interviewer asks you, "What is your strongest reaction to this dream?" After you answer, he or she asks, "What does that remind you of in your life?" Explore other strong reactions to dream characters, events, or objects with the same question: "What does that remind you of in your life?" Finally, your interviewer asks, "What do you feel the dream is trying to tell you?" After the "formal" questioning, you might want to hear your interviewer's reaction. Watch for any twinges of "a-ha" when he or she offers an opinion. Your visceral reaction is the most accurate way to gauge the truth of another's interpretation of your dream.

This is a wonderful tool to use with your partner, children, and parents. Sharing dreams and gathering meanings can offer solutions to problems. It can also help your family gain a better understanding of your pregnancy and help you understand your mate's or children's experience.

Self-portrait of Pregnancy

This self-portrait exercise is offered as a way to give expression to the multitude of feelings you may be having about being pregnant. It was inspired by Adriana Diaz's book, *Freeing the Creative Spirit*. You will briefly need someone to help you. This project unfolds best over a number of days, weeks, or even a month or more.

Start by making an outline of your body. Tape a piece of butcher paper slightly longer and wider than you to the floor. Lie down. Spend a few minutes trying out different positions until you find one that feels right. Call your helper in and have him or her trace your body with a pencil. When your outline is finished, hang it on a wall or door.

Next, consider the questions below while studying your outline.

1. What do I celebrate about my body during this pregnancy? What physical changes am I most in awe of? What have I loved about this experience so far?

2. What do I hate or resent about my body during this pregnancy? What part(s) of my body am I most afraid will hurt or fail me during labor?

3. What do I like about myself? What qualities will I be happy to pass on to my child?

4. What don't I like about myself? What are my fears about being a mother?

5. Spiritually, how do I feel right now? Have I had any insights since I've been pregnant?

6. What powerful or haunting dream images about pregnancy can I remember?

7. How do I feel about my baby? What hopes and visions do I have?

8. What images and feelings do I relate to being a mother?

9. How am I feeling about my own mother right now? What would I like to tell her if I could?

After rolling the questions around for a while, gather your art materials. Some people search for very specific items; others gather whatever sparks an "a-ha." You will need nontoxic glue and water-based paints and brushes, or colored pencils, crayons, or markers: whatever is affordable and handy. Old photos, magazine photos, newspaper captions, cotton balls, flower petals, branches, feathers, sequins, and fabric pieces are ideas of found objects that might help your self-portrait come alive.

Now, fill in your outline by expressing your feelings and images about your body, your baby, and your impending motherhood. Let the questions and materials inspire you but not oppress you: forget about getting it right or getting it done. Instead, lose yourself in making a full-sized image of the inner, pregnant you.

Questions 2, 4, and 9 are meant to evoke ideas for healing changes. For example, if you fear tearing your perineum during labor, on that area of your body you could draw a lotus blossom opening or glue an open, dried rose. If you've had a lot of nausea, you could draw healing symbols over your stomach. You can evoke a feeling of thankfulness and praise for your body by decorating your favorite parts. Your womb area can be filled with visualizations of what you hope and wish for your baby. Don't forget the border on the outside of your outline; you can fill that with prayers for yourself, your baby, your mate—anything!

Your portrait makes a great baby room or labor room decoration, or if you are shy, hang it on the inside of your closet or bedroom door.

Find a Beauty Spot

Go on a hunt for a "personal fount of beauty" near where you live or work. Places to seek include art museums, art galleries, craft stores, vistas, a trail through the woods, churches, cathedrals, public gardens, historic buildings, rivers and streams, lakes, and the ocean. The idea is to locate a stunning or ethereal or inspiring or exquisite or calming spot that you can visit easily. Margot found a soothing spot in a museum near a Dutch painting of two women attending a birth. Mia found a tiny waterfall in an enclosed, almost cavernlike area on a trail near her home. Sidney found walking through the historical section of Savannah gave her a sense of connection to all the women who had given birth before her. "I would read the date plates on different houses and imagine their lives." Lucia, who did not belong to a church or practice a religion, went for a drive after work one day and found a tiny wooden church with "scrubbed pine floors and a plain pulpit" about ten minutes off her regular commute. "I would visit this church every week, usually around sunset. I would just sit near the back and breathe. There were always flowers on the altar, but I never met anyone. I was always alone in this nourishing place." Visit your spot when you need a beauty fix, when you are worried, stressed, neglecting yourself, and after the baby comes, when you can't stand to have your nipple gnawed on one more time.

Resources:

Finding What You Didn't Lose: Expressing Your Truth and Creativity Through Poem-Making, by John Fox (Jeremy Tarcher, 1995). Lots of guidance for writing poetry for emotional well-being and healing.

Mother to Be's Dream Book: Understanding the Dreams of Pregnancy, by Raina M. Paris (Warner Books, 2000). Includes exercises to increase dream awareness and a glossary of common dream symbols as they pertain to pregnancy.

Move Your Stuff, Change Your Life How to Use Feng Shui to Get Love, Money, Respect and Happiness, by Karen Rauch Carter (Fireside, 2000). Some cheesy humor but I like this book because much of Feng Shui seems ways too serious for me.

No More Second Hand Art, by Peter London (Shambhala, 1989). Now a classic in the field of awakening creativity for adults.

With Child: Wisdom and Traditions for Pregnancy, Birth and Mothering, by Deborah Jackson (Chronicle Books, 1999). Filled with poetic musings and facts on what it means to become a mother, the mystery of pregnancy and birth, and the challenges of early motherhood.

The Spiritual Sustenance
of Pregnancy

When to Do It:

- When you need spiritual comfort and support for your pregnancy experience.

- If you are possessed by an extraordinary yearning to wrap your arms around the world and squeeze it tight.

- If you want to explore the spiritual power of pregnancy but don't know where to start or are afraid that by doing so, you will be dishonoring women who choose not to be mothers or be stretching the limits of your chosen religion.

What Is It?

Pregnancy is a numinous and magical state. It is a time when the barrier between the conscious and unconscious realms thins. It is a time to feel the presence of another soul developing alongside your own. It is a time when inner voices offer wise counsel louder and more clearly than usual, when we become aware that life is a continuum, when a woman may experience a bodily sense that *everything* around her is alive. Our connection to the cellular mystery of life is vibrantly stark and immediate. When you are pregnant, the polite and restrictive masks of everyday life that we have each created to survive can be stripped away, and you are immersed in the very juice of existence. No matter how many pictures of fetuses you look at or how many scientific facts you ingest, pregnancy remains a stunning, not-quite-possible-to-grasp marvel, a naked connection to the enigma of life. You can't escape the awe—and why would you want to?

You'll Need:

Clay, either non-firing or low firing.

A little time each day to be still.

Cardboard box, small shelf, or tabletop.

Objects that evoke good feelings about pregnancy and birth.

However, the great wonder of pregnancy is not to be confused with the archaic belief that motherhood is the ultimate fulfillment for a woman. We do not need pregnancy to give our existence meaning, to fulfill our biological destiny. Instead, pregnancy and birth are one of many alternatives we have the right to choose, one of many paths to spiritual understanding and creativity.

When we feel the power of life, both stirring within and burgeoning outside of us, we tend to treat ourselves, and others, with just a tad more reverence. Self-hatred becomes more difficult. Hating our enlarged bodies seems silly and we don't have as much patience for it. Worship of women's role in life readies us for being parents or strengthens our abilities if we already are. Finally, all of these ideas release stress and put us in touch with the bigger picture, always helpful, but especially important when we are pregnant.

What to Do:

Investigating Your Spiritual Perceptions

The women who helped me write this book spoke about how being pregnant had connected them to the cycle of life. When asked if pregnancy had been a spiritual experience, here is how some women responded:

> "How grand it is to be a woman!"
>
> Nancy Smith

> "Pregnancy is one of the great payoffs of being a woman—you get to grow this baby inside of you!"
>
> Marilyn

> "I'm more aware of the reality of death and the fleetingness of life, and how really precious my time is with my child."
>
> Susan

> "I have felt a strong power coming from my belly and in my meditations. I feel something in addition to my own spiritual senses."
>
> Marnee Shellabarger

"It gets you in touch with how magnificent the human body is. It's such a miracle, especially thinking how my first child was once inside of me, less than two years ago, and seeing what a miracle she is to behold now."

Lynne

"The ordinary earthiness surprised me. Pregnancy has felt so normal and right. I expected some sense of glamour or weirdness."

Susie

"I feel so connected to my purpose in life—the whole mother earth, Madonna thing. I feel so special because I know I am doing such an important thing by being a mother. I feel so blessed by being given this opportunity."

Lorie Helman

"I was supporting my father's frail body against mine. I saw myself, in the prime of life, and my baby inside me, at the very beginning of creation, and my father, about to die; I saw the whole picture of life."

Mary

Take a moment to reflect on how pregnancy has been a spiritual experience for you. What, if anything, has shifted in your perceptions of life? What are you aware of that you weren't before? Have you experienced any reverent moments in the course of your daily life? Or, for that matter, any irreverent moments? Avalon called herself a goddess bringing forth life, even as "I'm throwing up, corn chips are crunching under foot, Linnea's drawing on the wall, and there is barf on my forehead." What aren't you getting, in terms of spiritual nourishment, that you feel you need? Identify your longings, no matter how vague, and decide on one action you can take to meet a hunger.

Contemplating the Ancient Celebration of Birth

The earliest known images from prehistory are found in the innermost sanctuary of a cavern in Pech-Merle, France. The images are of pregnant women, one with a bird head, one headless, both intertwined with animals. Author and healer Vicki Noble notes, "The iconography of fertility worship was conjoined thirty thousand years ago with shamanic attributes. . . . At that time preparation to give birth did not imply confinement; on the contrary, it led to a joyous abandonment, a dance of life, a rapturous journey into the spirit world on the occasion of an intensely physical experience. . . ." A bit different from our current view of birth!

Throughout prehistory, statues, bas reliefs, and paintings of fertile women giving birth have been among the most numerous relics found. Tombs and sanctuaries were constructed to resemble a woman's body, with entrances through the birth canal. Even bread ovens were modeled after wombs. Compare this affirmation of fertility to the observation by artist Judy Chicago that for two thousand years there had been no images in Western art of women giving birth (until she originated her *Birth Project* in the early 1980s). A cornucopia of positive pregnancy and birth imagery existed in prehistoric times because birth mattered; ancient peoples recognized pregnancy as a momentous, mystical experience, each birth unique, each worthy of commemoration and celebration. To integrate the wisdom of the past, try these ideas:

Create your own birthing statue from clay. For inspiration, check out images from Elinor Gadon's *The Once and Future Goddess* or Marija Gimbutas's *The Language of the Goddess*. Kristina created clay images of women almost every month of her pregnancy, each one depicting how she was feeling that month about her experience. One figurine had stringy hair and tired eyes to reflect her exhaustion, another was the "leaf lady" to express her state of dreamy introspection. Jayne created a foot-high "round lady," which she had fired by a local potter and used to inspire her during labor. "It took quite awhile to come. I am not good with crafts, but I had this yearning to work with clay. I played with it for several weeks, making a mess. Finally, I just got out of the way by concentrating on the power of all the women who gave birth before me. I kept thinking about that instead of what my hands couldn't do. My statue wouldn't win any art contests, but she comforted me so much, before, during, and after birth!" Focus not on making something representational or beautiful, but on letting your unconscious have its say. If nothing recognizable emerges, fine. Simply enjoy the feel of the smooth, cool clay on your hands. (If you wish to make something that can be fired, be sure to knead or "wedge" the clay you are using for five to ten minutes before sculpting. This gets rid of the air bubbles and helps keep it from exploding in the kiln.)

Periodically, imagine yourself living in a prehistoric time when pregnant women and new mothers were revered. How would your perception of your experience be different if in the lobby of your office building or built in to the wall near the ATM you use there was a shrine filled with statues of ample women with pendulous breasts? (It is a hilarious idea, but also a tantalizing one.) Or if on the way home from work, you could stop at a temple where you would be treated as a goddess because you are pregnant? You might be enveloped in soft robes, your feet massaged with rare oils, your mind soothed by fragrant incense. Sure beats coming home to a cross toddler, nothing in the refrigerator, and work left over from the office! Tease your imagination before you go to bed at night or when you are riding a crowded bus home and no one offers you a seat. After a few imaginative forays, ask yourself, "If I lived in this time, how would I act differently? Would I feel any different about my growing body, my exhaustion, my ambivalence? If I lived in a world that honored women and children, how would my life be different?" You may find these short imaginative journeys bring with them a powerful dream, the need to pray or meditate, to dance, to visit a sacred place in nature, to write a story about how your life would be different, or to take some kind of political action like negotiating a better maternity leave policy for yourself. Go for it!

*See Work: Negotiating
Your Maternity Leave.*

Celebrating Your Connection to Life

Pregnancy shoots a big hole in the illusion that we are each separate people, encased in our own sphere of flesh, separated from the earth, from the animals, from the rocks, the ocean, the plants. Pregnancy allows you to palpably experience the permeability of life. Experiment with the ideas below.

Walk alone in nature as often as you can. Forget about getting your heart rate up or keeping your thighs taut. Instead, meander, look up, study the ground. Contemplate the fact that everything around you and inside of you is alive. Visualize your baby growing as you stroke a weathered rock, immerse your feet in a cold, gushing stream, lean against a canyon wall, or float down a river. Make the connection: my baby is alive; this rock (stream, river, patch of dirt, plant) is alive.

Sit in nature and imagine your skin is like a soft eggshell, permeable, with oxygen and other gases from the environment coming in and your own essence flowing out. Study your immediate vicinity. Pick one object—a tree, a pine needle, a nearby mountain. Imagine this object's "skin" is also like an eggshell, also permeable. Visualize the essence of this being traveling out of its "skin" to you and entering your "eggshell" and your essence doing the same. Practice this with different things in your environment.

See I Want My Mommy:
Mothering Yourself.

Lie on the Earth in a sheltered spot—under a little rock overhang, in a bed of moss, under a big tree. Close your eyes and breathe. Sink into the Earth. Let her support you. Breathe. When you feel relaxed and peaceful, focus on the baby in your womb. Visualize him or her there, inside of you, depending on you for oxygen, nourishment, safety. Visualize yourself looking down at you from far above, lying on the Earth. Visualize the Earth as your womb, feeding you, protecting you, giving you food. Visualize the people you love. See them being fed from this living planet. Finally, spend a few moments thinking about what gifts your baby has given you so far—how by depending on you, your child-to-be has already helped you grow. Then consider what you have given to the Earth, how you have helped her grow, how the planet benefits by having you on her surface.

Exploring the Values You Want to Impart

Pregnancy is preparation for parenting. Pregnancy offers nine months to switch gears, to shed outmoded parts of yourself and dust off any meaningful values you might have let slip into the background of your life. You might find yourself attending the church of your childhood for the first time in twenty years. Or you might find yourself yearning for new spiritual traditions and rituals, wanting to create ones without painful attachments to the past. Great. What you don't want to do is unconsciously mimic or reject your parents' values. If you reject your parents' ways without trying to understand, love, or at least forgive their traditions, you set yourself up to play out the same patterns and to confront similar conflicts with your child(ren). Conversely, if you follow your family traditions without stopping to ask yourself if these truly feed your spiritual needs, you may find yourself (or your child) in a spiritual crisis later in life. Use this time to consciously consider, alone and if necessary with your mate, what your values and beliefs are. Even if you are very active in a religion, it is still wonderful to talk about your beliefs and concerns. Having a child gives you the initiative to consider the big questions: What is the meaning of my life? What values do I want to impart to my child? What rituals and traditions do I wish our family to celebrate? What did my parents teach me that I want to pass on?

It is not uncommon for conflicts to arise at this time between your mate and you, but also with your parents, your mate's parents, even brothers and sisters. Couples may suddenly find themselves fighting over the meaning of Christmas, over joining a church, or over one partner's spiritual beliefs. Because most of us don't spend much time verbalizing our spiritual beliefs, either to ourselves or our partner, pregnancy can conjure up a lot of hard-to-answer questions that you may have only vaguely touched on before. Start early in the pregnancy to discuss these. If the conversation gets heated, ask yourself, "Why do I (or why does my partner) have such an emotional attachment to this idea or tradition?" Don't fixate on getting your way or winning; that style of parental decision making wears thin fast. Try to view the other person's ideas with acceptance or at least tolerance. Write about your beliefs and share this with each other.

Strengthening Your Intuition

It just so happens that the most essential act of self-nurturing is also the most essential act of good mothering (and healthy pregnancy): taking enough quiet time each day to check in with yourself. As many women reported to me, "When I listen to my inner wisdom, I know how to be a good mother. I know what I need to do."

The biggest hurdle separating you from your inner wisdom is slowing down enough to hear it. Pregnancy helps in this arena because you often find yourself needing to nap, rock, unwind, or just be more than usual. Use this time to develop your intuition. Use this time to see what you know that you haven't had time to process. To see what your body needs that you haven't had time to give it. To see where you have gotten off-track. This kind of quiet self-reflection is almost impossible with a dependent infant or bustling toddler, but if you practice now, it will be easier to slip into this intuitive state in the five minutes you grab for a shower, the time you need to poop, the few still moments before sleep. If you already have a dependent infant, it becomes even more important—and even more impossible—to check in with yourself, to honor your wisdom. Try to take five minutes when the child is asleep to meditate or sit quietly. Tell yourself it's more important than returning your cousin's phone call, ordering that wedding gift, or reading the paper. But if you can't, forget about it. A sense of failing will block your intuition faster than a double margarita.

Establish a Reminder

Create a pregnancy and birth shrine to inspire you to take care of yourself, nurture your spirit, to slow down and put your pregnancy first for at least a few minutes daily. I bought a small shelf and put it in my bedroom, where I arranged icons and images that inspired me. When the birth grew near, I added positive notes about how my body could do it, a small birthing goddess I made (see page 194), and a postcard of an open lotus blossom. To construct your shrine, pick a shelf or tabletop in a private corner. Or construct a small triptych (three panels with a floor, like a small stage) from a cardboard box. Paint or decorate the box, and you have a portable shrine you can take to the hospital with you. (Who cares if the staff thinks you're weird? It's *your* birth.)

Decorate your shrine with images of pregnancy, birth, and mothering that whisper positive, divine messages to you; mementos that link you to other birthing women, especially in your own family; spiritual comforters like a statue of Mary or a small book of poetry. Find shrine articles by checking card stores, museum catalogs, funky gift shops, and stores that specialize in nature goodies, by rummaging through your treasures, or by looking for pleasing objects on a rocky slope, in a thatch of woodlands, or on a busy city street.

Make Time for a Retreat

Another common thread that emerged during research for this project was how many women, even second-time moms, had made time for a spiritual retreat of some kind during their pregnancies. Diane visited a spa with her best friend, participating in soulful conversation, hours of yoga, early morning hikes, and healthful food. Mary spent a silent meditation weekend at a Zen monastery. "I had a whole chunk of time to myself with no phones, no demands; the monks cooked these delicious meals, it really fed me." (A common theme on spiritual retreats for pregnant women seems to be good food prepared by someone else!) The possibilities are endless, and the reasons to do it *now* include:

- You won't have much time for yourself for quite a while.

- Labor and delivery are very demanding experiences. A good inner rest can be invaluable.

- You are more emotionally and intuitively sensitive and can gain wonderful insights.

- You deserve it!

Resources:

Celebrating Motherhood: A Comforting Companion for Every Expecting Mother, by Andrea Alban Gosline, Lisa Burnett Bossi, and Ame Mahler Beanland (Conari Press/Red Wheel Weiser, 2001). Inspiring!

Joyful Birth: A Spiritual Path to Motherhood (Includes 2 CDs) compiled by Susan Piver (Rodale, 2002). Helpful, well-written essays from different experts on spirituality and parenting and 2-CD's containing simple yoga instruction, aromatherapy suggestions, journaling exercises, meditations, and soothing music (classical).

10 Principles for Spiritual Parenting: Nurturing Your Child's Soul, by Mimi Doe and Marsh Walch (Perennial, 1998). How to honor your children's natural spirituality.

What's Going to Happen to Me After the Baby Is Born?

You'll Need:

Your journal or paper, and a pen.

When to Do It:

- When you're having dreams of forgetting or losing your baby.

- When you feel ambivalent, resentful, or nothing at all toward the baby or your body.

- If you aren't allowing yourself to change your lifestyle to reflect your pregnancy.

- If you are afraid June Cleaver, Mrs. Robinson, or Madame Bovary will arise from the delivery bed.

What Is It?

Do you wonder and worry about the changes a baby will bring to your personal identity? Will you be reduced to one big breast? How many of the things you identify as *you* will disappear after the baby arrives? *Every woman worries that her identity will be changed in ways she will regret.*

This was my greatest fear about childbirth. I was worried about disappearing forever into a cloud of baby demands with no time for my own creativity. Eighteen years later, I would reemerge, but it would be too late. Nothing would be left of the Jennifer we knew (the people I drive crazy might like that). In her place would be a washed-out, sagging-breasted, boring mother. I needed to construct a new paradigm, a vision of mothering that included seeing myself making mud pies, driving carpool, reassuring nighttime fears *and* writing books, making love, leading canoe trips.

My fears were not unfounded. The passage into motherhood bears a striking resemblance to puberty. During adolescence, your vision of yourself slips and slides through dramatic physical, emotional, and mental changes. Disequilibrium is the norm. Pregnancy can be equally unsettling. Part of you is in chrysalis, waiting to emerge as a mother. A mother! A new and utterly foreign identity—even for second-times moms, who must integrate the unknown reality of being a mother to two (or more) children. *Having a child entails a fundamental change in your selfhood, a major and unalterable shift.* Having a baby requires changes in your lifestyle (to state the obvious) but, more significantly, changes in your psyche. It does require sacrifice. It is worth it. There is nothing like the smell of your baby's sweet milky breath or the way her head feels like a firm, fuzzy peach in your hand. *But motherhood does not require that you or your needs cease to exist.* Being a self-less mother entails disconnecting from yourself until you wake up at your child's high school graduation and don't know who you are. Being a self-ful mother means you forge the difficult path of balancing your needs with your child(ren)'s, creating a dynamic portrait of a woman who loves her children and has a life of her own.

It is extraordinarily difficult to maintain any sense of yourself when baby is screaming for you, your partner wants to have sex (and you feel guilty because you would rather read or sleep), you have a long list of phone calls to return, and the laundry pile is so high that walking past it is life threatening. But if you can put yourself first right now and use the liminal state of pregnancy to forge a commitment to protect and nourish your authentic self, you are more likely to weather the changes in your self-image and to enjoy the experience of merging with your infant.

What To Do:

Exploring Your Changing Identity

The transition time of pregnancy provides an invitation to explore your changing identity. These exercises are not meant to produce a neat or psychologically definitive picture of who you are. Rather, they may help you appreciate yourself as you are now, anticipate some of the changes to your identity, and pinpoint some of the aspects of your-self that will not change. These exercises are best done quickly and when you will not be disturbed. For women who are already moms, that might be early in the morning or locked in the bathroom. As always, nothing offered here is meant to overwhelm or depress you. Sample only what you have energy for.

Title a piece of paper "Parts of My Life I Like Best." List everything that comes to mind. Be honest with yourself; don't include activities or people because you are supposed to. A writing technique to use if you feel stuck is to set a timer for five minutes and keep writing until the timer goes off.

Entitle another sheet "Parts of My Self I Most Fear Losing." What do you fear will disappear when you become a mother? It may be noth-ing, it may be something tiny or hard to define. Give this topic five minutes' thought.

Next, construct a list for "What I Think I Will Gain in My Life." This is the space to anticipate the extravagant happiness, the exclusive love relationship, the total engrossment of having a child. Consider too how baby will help you grow as a person.

Finally, make a list of "Parts of My Life I Don't Mind Losing." Here is the place to think about how you can simplify your life, what sacri-fices you are consciously willing to make to create room for your new child. Don't be dismayed if this list is the shortest. The process of rear-ranging and stripping down your life takes place after the baby becomes a reality. This is just a warm-up.

Use the lists as a jumping-off point for action. For instance:

Take one aspect you like about your life and celebrate it, make it larger, do it more often. (One of mine was buying books—a dangerous one to do more often!) Or a favorite friend you long to spend time with—carve out a weekend to hole up and gossip together (or at least have a long phone conversation).

Ruminate on the parts of your self you are most afraid of losing. Ask yourself, "Why am I afraid of losing this part of myself?" Or ask yourself, "What can I do to sustain this part of myself?" This kind of questioning is best done gently and slowly, nibbling tenderly around the edges of your psyche.

Don't forget what you think you'll gain in your life. This is a good one to share with your mate or birth partner, a friend who is already a mother, or your mother.

"Parts of My Life I Don't Mind Losing" is an early blueprint for simplifying your life to reflect your changing concerns and interests. Brainstorm one or two actions to take prebaby. If one of the things you wouldn't mind losing is huge, like your job or your house mortgage, proceed slowly! The urge to simplify can be heady.

Postpartum

Reread these lists six months postpartum, then again when your child is eighteen months or so old. Would you change anything now?

Affirm Your Sense of Self

The best insurance against losing your self is to spend time during your pregnancy exploring and affirming who you are and what you take pleasure in. The more you appreciate and accept yourself now, the less you will try to be a perfect mother to prove your worth. Try these ideas:

Ask yourself, "What do I want to do for just me?" Compose a wish list. Give yourself as many of these treats as you can. My list was: Restart therapy, write fiction, go live in a cabin by myself in Big Sur, have girlfriends over for a slumber party, go canoeing, go camping with Chris, scoop up the world and plunge my arms into its fertile wildness (I made my list late at night). Obviously, unless you aren't working and have deep financial resources, you won't be able to do everything on your list. But *please* push yourself to do the most cherished items, especially the ones that will be difficult to do once baby arrives.

Create or buy a reminder of who you are prebaby. It could be a framed photo of you scaling Mount Everest, a rose quartz necklace to symbolize your inner life, a rock from a lake you loved as a child. Display it prominently.

Do things that give you a sense of mastery. Making a flourless chocolate torte, taking a pottery class, growing an ordered row of sunflowers—whatever makes you feel confident.

Cats are supposed to have nine lives. If you could live eight other lives besides the one you are living right now, what would you do? Mine are shaman, Jungian analyst, rich art collector, vagabond, hermit, and painter. Make a quick list of your imaginary lives. Have fun. Inspired by your list, pick one or two things to do that make your pulse quicken or your ears perk up. Mine could be take a shamanism workshop, visit an art gallery and pretend to be able to afford the art, or drive up the coast by myself and camp out.

See Nurturing Yourself
During Pregnancy: If You
Could . . . for another
pleasure-exploring
exercise.

Answer the question "If I didn't feel it were too selfish, what would I do for myself?" This question gets right to the heart of what you might do for yourself if you felt no pressure to be good or nice or nurture others first. Dare to fulfill your wildest longings now.

Reconnect with Childhood

Reconnecting with enchanting parts of our childhood is especially touching when pregnant. A sad feeling associated with giving birth is knowing you will no longer be only a daughter to your parents, you will have to share your mate's affection, and you will finally have to grow up (at least a little). Soften this change from daughter to mother, from child to parent by remembering the part of yourself that is still a child.

Relax somewhere quiet and travel back to a prepuberty age when you were happy and felt good about yourself. Allow pleasant memories, refreshing sensations, feelings to bubble up. Take your time; don't worry about pulling something specific into memory, just drift. If it appeals to you, write a letter with your nondominant hand (the hand you don't usually write with) from this little girl to the pregnant woman you are today. What does this little girl know that would help you make this transition and still retain your "girl" wisdom and centering?

Think of three traits you liked in yourself as a child. How can you bring one of those characteristics into your life today? For instance, if honesty is one, who can you be truly honest with today?

Name what your child self doesn't want to give up by becoming a mother. Being number one to your mate, being the center of attention at family gatherings, getting lots of Christmas presents—nothing is too petty. Consider grieving if that feels appropriate.

See Ambivalence: Grieving the Changes.

Reflect on what you might need from your father now—a long hug and the reassurance you will always be his little girl; a lunch alone together; a fierce game of Scrabble and hot chocolate; a frank discussion about what it was like to be a father; or a conversation about becoming a grandfather. If your father is deceased or you are estranged from him (physically or emotionally), acknowledge what you wish your father could give you during this pregnancy. Give yourself time to mourn the reality that he cannot.

See I Want My Mommy for help getting what you need from your mother.

The Myth of the Perfect Mother: Exploring Cultural Baggage

Icon, archetype, upholder of moral values, Eve, Virgin Mary, Aunt Jemima, Donna Reed, a safe haven, a warm lap, existing only for children, above all a font of unconditional love and acceptance—no other identity is so fraught with emotion, history, and projections of other people's unconscious desires and conflicts than the role of mother.

Adrienne Rich wrote, in *Of Woman Born,* about her first pregnancy at age twenty-six:

> I realize I was effectively alienated from my real body and my real spirit by the institution—not the fact—of motherhood. This institution—the foundation of human society as we know it— allowed me only certain views, certain expectations, whether embodied in the booklet in my obstetrician's waiting room, the novels I had read, my mother-in-law's approval, my memories of my own mother, the Sistine Madonna or she of Michelangelo's Pietà, the floating notion that a woman pregnant is a woman calm in her fulfillment or simply a woman waiting.

The potent and damaging myth of the perfect mother has become woven into our belief systems like fishing line: invisible but nearly unbreakable. This myth is an unattainable absolute that tells us our children are exceptionally fragile creatures completely at the mercy of our imperfections and mistakes, that the way our children turn out is solely our responsibility (the dominant culture has nothing to do with it), and above all, the perfect mother is someone who always loves her child unconditionally and is always absolutely fulfilled by mother-hood. Is it any wonder mothers are bewildered and self-conscious, hounded by guilt, haunted by how much more we should be doing? Is it any wonder we feel ambivalent about becoming mothers? *How can we ever measure up?* We must liberate ourselves from this myth by examining our own expectations and associations.

Explore your associations with motherhood through clustering, a writing technique pioneered by Gabriele Rico. In the middle of a piece of paper, write *mother* and draw a circle around it. With the word *mother* acting as a stimulus, let go and quickly record all the associations that spring into your mind, using one word or short phrases. Write quickly, without editing, encasing each word in its own circle, radiating outward from the center in any direction that feels right. Connect each word or phrase with a line to the preceding circle. When something new occurs to you, begin again at *mother* and radiate outward until that line of associations is exhausted. Keep going until you feel finished. Read your web. Are there any surprises? Any associations you want to explore further? Any trouble spots of perfection to watch out for?

Rummage through the scrap heap of cultural beliefs and expectations about mothering so that you can become conscious of what you wish to keep and what you wish to discard. You might want to discuss the following questions with a pregnant friend, your mother, your partner, or write free-form answers in your journal. Or postpartum, explore with a group of new mothers:

- What are your expectations for yourself as a mother? Some thoughts will float to the surface quickly, others will take time. Ruminate on this one. Peer into your assumptions.

- Name a few characteristics of an *ideal* mother.

- If you could, would you be this ideal mother? What would have to change in your life and your personality?

- Name a fictional role model that has influenced your idea of motherhood. Perhaps an actress who seems to effortlessly manage to balance being perfectly fit with having three kids? Or a mother you read about as a child in a novel?

- Scrutinize your environment for images of mothers. Scan parenting magazines in your health care provider's office. Watch TV shows, movies, advertising images. What do these images say? How do they make you feel?

- Does a mother have to be selfless? How would you define selfless?

- In the first three months, what would make you see yourself as failing to be a good mother? Going back to work, not breast-feeding, not loving every moment?

For the next few days, as you live your life, ask yourself, "What parts of my life don't fit with my image of being a mother?" Dig below the surface to find your beliefs about what a mother does, what her life looks like. An example from my pregnant life was driving a little fast on the freeway at sunset listening to loud rock 'n' roll. I thought to myself, "Once the baby is here, I can't do this anymore." Underneath I believed I could never act that way again. Other examples might include having boisterous sex or initiating sex, wearing fashionable or revealing clothes, reading trashy novels, or having a romantic late dinner. True, you might not have the time, energy, or resources to do some of these things. That is not the issue. The issue is, Would you allow yourself to still enjoy them?

You yearn to be kind, patient, giving, to be an excellent role model to your child(ren). When you make mistakes, you feel guilty. This kind of guilt signals where you need to grow as a mother, is short-lived, and is healthy. But the daily, energy-sapping guilt that plagues so many of us is damaging, unproductive, and fueled by this culturally engineered myth of the perfect mother. We can never measure up, so we will always feel terrible. By obliterating this myth, shame and mothers can part ways for good.

Resources:

A Life's Work: On Becoming a Mother, by Rachel Cusk (Picador, 2003). Unsentimental, dry, honest, and rather grim at times—good for those who are struggling and want to feel less alone.

Buddha Never Raised Kids and Jesus Didn't Drive Carpool: Seven Principles for Parenting With Soul, by Vickie Falcone (Jodere Group, June 2003). Positive, practical, spiritual, parenting guidance.

Diary of a Mother: Parenting Stories and Other Stuff, by Christine Louise Hohlbaum (iUniverse, June 2003). Recommended by a reader who loved it.

I Wish Someone Had Told Me: A Realistic Guide to Early Motherhood, by Nina Barrett. (Academy Chicago Publishers, 1997)

Mother Journeys: Feminists Write About Mothering, edited by Maureen T. Reddy, Martha Roth, Amy Sheldon, T. Reddy (Spinster's Ink, 1994). Stories, poems, cartoons, essays, and more by feminist mothers.

Mother Shock: Loving Every (Other) Minute of It, by Andrea Buchanan (Seal Press, 2003). A painfully honest, funny, and compassionate look at the culture shock of life as a new mother.

Of Woman Born, by Adrienne Rich (New York: Norton, 1976). Rich's often-quoted, brilliant work remains fascinating and thought provoking.

The Big Rumpus: A Mother's Tale from the Trenches, by Ayun Halliday (Seal Press, 2001). The new Erma Bombeck—funny, honest, evocative.

Preparing
for Postpartum

When to Do It:

- Starting anytime you feel the urge but at least three or four weeks before your due date, if possible.

- If you decide to spend some time with a friend who has a new baby and end up sobbing on the floor of her bathroom because you can't believe what you've gotten yourself into.

- If planning and organizing make you feel nurtured and safe.

What Is It?

Pregnancy is like a new romance: it doesn't have a lot to do with reality, you don't give much concrete thought to the future, you feel very special, and you exist in your own little world. Pregnancy ends with birth. Most of us give only vague thought to what happens after that. *This is a big mistake.* But it's almost unavoidable, because you can't fully imagine what your life is going to be like with a baby. (This is true for the second or third child as well. Mothers reported that the adjustment from zero to one was easier than the adjustment from one to two. Others reported that the adjustment from one to two was nothing, but going from two to three drove them wild.)

We anticipate, strategize, train for the birth but give little thought to what we will do after this climax. *But postpartum preparation is as important as birth preparation.* From examining your expectations to arranging a detailed support plan, the more prepared you are for the emotionally wild, woolly, wonderful, and physically draining months

You'll Need:

A variety of mommy-centered postpartum supplies—from food you can eat cold to a chair with excellent back support.

Tons of support from loving, non-critical friends and family.

The courage to look at your own expectations and defy the expectations others have of you.

following the arrival of your miracle baby, the better you will able to mother your infant and yourself. You will also be less likely to suffer needlessly from illness, depression, or breast-feeding problems, and you will be more able to enjoy and learn from this glorious and sometimes harrowing transformation.

What to Do:

I Didn't Know What to Expect

Too many women are needlessly shocked and irate over the lack of information they receive about how their lives are going to change. Time and time again I heard, "I had no idea" or "I'm so angry that nobody told me" or "Why doesn't anybody talk about the bad stuff?" I think there are several reasons.

One, you probably don't want to hear it. It might even be making you angry to read this, to think that everything about your soon-to-arrive child won't always please and delight you. "No," you say, "I know it can be tough. But how tough can it really be?" We don't want to, and are perhaps incapable of, grasping the changes careening our way. We shut out or defuse any truths our friends with children try to impart. We think to ourselves, "They don't have the rock solid equal partnership we do" or "She is so disorganized" or "We have more money" or more support or a better sense of humor or whatever. "It will be different for us." And that is true—it will be different for you. *Having a can-do positive attitude is vital.* But it is also vital that you recognize things will change.

Also, words are often inadequate when you are trying to express the experience of nurturing a child. For example, one night when walking Lillian around the living room for the thousandth time, trying to get her to stop crying and start sleeping, I was bombarded with frustration, hopelessness, and self-loathing. But, literally sixty seconds later, when she fell asleep in my lap, I felt drenched with joy, marveling at these tiny, dimpled knees and tiny, round wrists that came out of me. You startle awake at the first whimper, hating to leave sleep but excited to hold your baby again. Daily reality becomes astonishing.

One day Lillian was sleeping in Chris's office. I ran into the kitchen and grabbed his hand. "Honey, come quick, there's a *baby* asleep in your office!" It can feel like winning the lottery, getting everything you wanted for Christmas, and falling in love all wrapped into one. It also feels like being marooned on a deserted arctic island in a blizzard, naked, with only Rush Limbaugh for company.

Another reason you may not feel informed is that people forget what the passage into parenthood was like. Their perspective changes. They move into a new area—teething, toddlers who won't share, schooling. Just as your parents may remember only the good stuff about raising you, your friends and family may forget the exposed and potent feelings, the fog-inducing exhaustion, the giddy enchantment, the ecstasy at a long nap or a well-timed poop. Or perhaps it is all a conspiracy and, as one woman said, "They lie."

So it may be just about impossible to grasp what life with baby will be like—both the incredible highs and the amazing lows. However, there are a few things you can do to smooth the transition.

Examine Your Expectations

Look over the questions in previous chapters having to do with expectations for how life will look after the baby arrives. It doesn't matter if you don't have a partner or your partner isn't interested; most of these questions still apply.

See Connecting with Your Partner: Examining Your Expectations; and What's Going to Happen to Me After the Baby Is Born?: The Myth of the Perfect Mother.

The point is not to overwhelm or depress yourself but to sketch a picture of what you imagine your postbaby life will look like. How realistic is your vision? What expectations do you have for yourself? One of the most important things you can do to prepare yourself for life after baby is to understand what you expect of yourself and to inquire of yourself what will happen if you don't meet your expectations. How will you cope? How will your partner cope?

If you have a partner, it is crucial you discuss the fact that you cannot be expected to do everything. It is equally crucial that you believe this yourself, that you start giving yourself permission now *not to do it alone* and *not to do it all perfectly.* Especially if you are single mom, you must

See Receiving the Nurturing You Need from Your Partner Postpartum for specific ideas.

find people you can rely on for help. If you have a partner, plan on your mate giving middle-of-the-night relief bottles *regularly* even if you are going to nurse (you can express milk and give a bottle starting from two to six weeks after the birth; check with your health care provider or pediatrician, since each baby is different). Talk about how you and your mate will get time to yourselves—alone and together—but know that before baby it is pretty impossible to anticipate exactly how things will fall together (or apart). Find baby-sitters and save money for this service now.

Hang out around new moms (you could attend a new mothers' group). Listen. Ask questions.

After you have considered your expectations and listened to other mothers, what do you still secretly, in your heart of hearts, expect the first few weeks and months with your baby to be like? What are you still expecting from yourself? For example, Dorothy thought she had a pretty realistic view of what life would be like because it was her second child, but when she dug deep enough, she realized she was positive her second baby would be easier than her first (a comforting myth), and that because her first child was five there would be no problem with sibling rivalry. "I pictured all three of us snuggled together in bed and myself always calm and able to smooth things over. I realized how unrealistic I might be when I saw a friend's six-year-old whack her one-year-old brother on the head." Do yourself a favor: plumb the depths of your expectations.

Cocoon

When a baby is on the way, most of the energy goes into preparing his or her room and gathering baby supplies. But you also need to give thought to your needs, to what you can do now to create a more comfortable transition into motherhood.

If you don't have one, buy or borrow an answering machine. This becomes a very important postbaby tool when you simply cannot or must not answer the phone.

A portable phone or long cord on a phone is another handy sanity tool.

Buy two boxes of the largest sanitary pads available. If you normally wear cotton pads that you wash, buy at least one box of disposable, because you might find yourself without any time to wash them out. Have one box of medium-sized pads on hand too.

Stock up on foods that comfort you as well as food you can eat quickly and with one hand. Toaster pastries from the health food store, low-fat frozen yogurt, trail mix, cheese and crackers, energy drinks, rice cakes, and (especially) cookies work well.

Stash away a few "treats" to pull out when you are feeling low, when you want to celebrate, or when you feel blobby and fat. Scented skin lotion, a new T-shirt, or a great book can lift your spirits a bit.

See Comforting Clothing and Other Sensual Strategies: Postnatal Wardrobe.

Make sure you have some comfy, loose clothes.

Good things to have on hand: a pitcher or a sports bottle with a flexible straw for water; things to put your hair in (hair bands, ties, even a hat); herbs and essential oils for sitz baths; thank-you notes or stationery; birth announcements made or ordered if you are doing them; hemorrhoid cream; prenatal vitamins (you will continue taking these); prune juice (if you get constipated); film (store in refrigerator to keep fresh); an easy-to-use camera; photo albums; baby advice books; extra basics like shampoo, toilet paper, and baby detergent; a plastic doughnut to sit on; stain remover; thick nursing pillow (a U-shaped neck pillow works great); lip balm; night lights (the kind that go off during the day—place in baby's room, your room, the hall, the bathroom and you'll be able to avoid turning on lights at night, which helps you and the baby get back to sleep faster).

See Appendix: Herbs, Oils, and Other Natural Comforters for sitz bath information.

See Resources for baby advice books.

If you are planning to nurse, have on hand several good nursing bras and some nursing pads. Cotton and washable pads are best, but because not every woman leaks, don't stock up yet; buy a small package of disposable pads for now. If you are returning to work and will continue to breast-feed, locate where you will rent or buy your pump now (ask your health care provider who in your area rents or sells breast pumps).

See Comforting Clothing and Other Sensual Strategies: Postnatal Wardrobe for bra guidelines.

See Resources.

If you are due for a haircut or teeth cleaning, get these done about two weeks before your due date.

Scan your calendar two to four months into the future for birthdays
and holidays. If you can, buy cards and gifts now. Then all you have to
do is mail or deliver.

Preparing to Breast-Feed

If you plan on breast-feeding, please, please take a class before the
birth. Breast-feeding is a *learned* art. You aren't born knowing how to
do it. Even animals in the wild must learn how to do it (by observing
others animals).

See Resources.

Buy or borrow several books on breast-feeding. Do not wait until after
the birth.

If possible, watch other mothers breast-feed. You can learn a lot by
observing.

Find out what kind of breast-feeding support is provided by your hospital, doctor, or midwife directly after the birth. You need someone
who *shows* you how, and you may need someone to show you how
more than once. If you are having your baby in a hospital and the
hospital doesn't provide help, you will want to have your own support
present. You also want to inquire how supportive your hospital is of
breast-feeding by asking your doctor or midwife what the hospital
policy is.

Do not assume that obstetricians know much about breast-feeding.
They might, but then again, they might not. One mother had inverted
nipples and didn't know it, even though she had been seeing her
OB/GYN for ten years. She ended up taking her baby to the hospital
with dehydration three times before a nurse in the emergency room
mentioned calling a lactation specialist. She was diagnosed over the
phone and immediately given the help she needed, ending a frustrating and dangerous nightmare. Moral of the story? Locate a good
breast-feeding helper *ahead of time* who can help you once you are
home. It is common for a mom to feel great about breast-feeding in
the hospital and then run into problems when her milk comes in or
exhaustion confuses things. You may need breast-feeding help several
times; Kristina needed five visits to work out her and Sam's difficulties.

You may need help weaning. You need someone you can phone almost any time. This person could be:

- A friend or relative with whom you feel very comfortable and who has breast-fed more than one child;

- A peer group like your local La Leche League;

- Your health care provider or a staff person at the hospital or birthing center you plan on using;

- A doula or birthing assistant;

- A lactation consultant—someone who has been trained in all aspects of routine and special-circumstance breast-feeding. Their training can be anywhere from "I breast-fed three children" to sitting for the International Lactation Consultant's Association licensing exam—the latter is best.

Find your helper by:

- Asking other women who breast-fed what their experience was like and who helped them;

- Asking your obstetrician, your pediatrician, or any of your local hospitals or birthing centers whom they recommend;

- Contacting the International Lactation Consultant's Association for a local referral;

See Resources.

- Contacting the La Leche League to see if there is a group or support person near you.

When choosing help, keep in mind that what you need is someone who is calm, reassuring, and will not give you piecemeal information. You also need someone who makes you feel comfortable with the physicalness of breast-feeding, hopefully someone you could ask just about anything. Finally, you need a helper who respects your needs and is not dogmatic.

If someone is volunteering to help, diplomatically find out what her experience is. How many moms has she volunteered with? How long has she been helping? How many babies has she breast-fed herself? What, if any, training does she have?

If you are hiring a lactation consultant, ask:

- What is her certification or the number of hours she has of lactation training?

- When is the last time she updated her training? (New information is being discovered regularly.)

- What is her availability? How soon can you see her?

- Does she have a back-up if she is not available?

- What does she charge? (It may be by the hour or by the visit. The first visit is usually more; the fees range widely and can be on a sliding scale.) There are excellent volunteer lactation consultants, including the La Leche League. Don't let lack of funds stop you from getting help.

See Postbirth
Nourishment: Surviving
and Thriving: Breast-
Feeding Comfort for more
details.

Decide where you will feed your baby. Eventually, you will just plop down and feed him or her anywhere, but in the beginning you will be putting all your energy into getting the positioning right, so it helps to have a comfortable, well-organized spot to reduce frustration.

Some babies simply do not know how to breast-feed. Trying to feed your newborn and not being able to tops the list of grim experiences. Starting at six weeks, Lillian rejected my breast; it turned out she was allergic to the dairy and corn I was eating. I felt she hated me; I felt rejected at the most primal level. Although it is superb to be deeply committed to breast-feeding (and necessary in American culture because breast-feeding is still not widely accepted), it is also important to be flexible so that if you run into complications, your entire self-esteem as a mother is not squashed. Like nonmedicated birth, breast-feeding has become the symbol of good mothering, and in the process, too many women are being made to feel inadequate and negligent if they cannot or choose not to. Remember my motto: every pregnancy, every child, every woman is unique. Trust yourself. You do know best.

Postbaby Support Plan

Ideally, what mothers should be able to have at this time is a self-styled sanctuary. A suspension of usual activity. A shower.

A massage. A comforting grandmother. An extra pair of hands. A stolen moment between cries or feedings for Mom and Dad to remember who they were and "try on" who they are now.

This is from Sally Placksin in her wonderful resource book, *Mothering the New Mother.* Get some paper and a pen. It is time to organize your sanctuary in writing—*precisely* who is going to nurture you postpartum. Don't worry if you can't fill in all the blanks or you feel exhausted when considering all the help you might need. These questions represent what would be perfect, but none of us lives in a perfect world. However, be careful if you have too many blanks; it is too easy to underestimate the amount of support you need.

When filling in these blanks, don't count on only one person to do most of the work, especially if this one person is your partner. He or she is also going through a monumental adjustment and also needs time alone and nurturing.

Don't rule out hiring help. Doulas, mothering-the-mother services, or professional postpartum services are increasingly popular as alternatives to traditional support. Doulas nurture you and free you to nurture your baby. "I'm not close with my mother and my sister doesn't have any children. Having a doula service not only allowed me to get rest and eat well, but it gave me other women to share this incredible experience with. I hired what women in other cultures have: a group of women to cuddle and support me. It was wonderful," noted Jackie, mother of Luke. What you want is someone to take care of you, not necessarily take care of the baby. Sarah's parents hired her a baby nurse. "I wanted to be alone with my baby. The nanny made me feel very awkward and unsure of my instincts. It wasn't until after she left that I finally started to feel like a mom." However, having a nurse or nanny at night who brings you the baby to feed, then burps, changes, and gets him or her back to sleep can be heaven, especially for single moms or moms with unsupportive mates. Whatever you decide, you want to avoid a helper who makes you feel intimidated or who overrides your ideas. Be sure to get fees in writing to avoid confusion later. Don't hesitate to ask if you can customize or shrink services. "I can't afford that. Could you do this?" is a perfectly acceptable question.

There are a few volunteer doula services or mothering mentors in some communities, especially for teen mothers. Check with your local birth center, church, synagogue, or hospital.

Fill in as many blanks as you can:

Obstetrician/midwife _____

Childbirth assistant or doula _____

Pediatrician _____

Breast-feeding support
person directly after birth _____

Breast-feeding support person at home
(doulas and midwives can usually provide this) _____

_____

Hospital or clinic warm-line number _____

New mothers' support group _____

Postpartum depression hot-line
number or local contact group or person _____

_____

Two to ten people over a two-week period who will bring meals, clean, watch older siblings, take out garbage, walk dog, do laundry, run errands, or watch baby so you can sleep. Note: Even if you are having someone come to stay or you have a devoted partner, arrange some outside help. It is too much for one person to do. If you are hiring a doula, you may need a little help after she is gone. Having these helpers lined up is *mandatory* for single moms. _____

_____

_____

If you have lots of friends and family,
designate one person to coordinate offers of help _____

_____

Baby-sitters for day and night (family, friends, plus people you hire)

_____

"Mother's helper" (preteen) to help while you are home _____

_____

Someone to call during the night to talk to when you don't
know what to do (especially important for single moms
or mothers whose partners travel a lot; could be the
number of a twenty-four-hour hospital warm line) _____

_____

Another new mother with whom you
can share the good and bad times _____

A neighbor you can call in an emergency (from watching the baby
for a half an hour while you shower to driving you to the hospital)

_____

Someone close to you to whom you could turn if you became
seriously depressed or had an anxiety attack (this should be
someone you feel very comfortable with and who is somewhat
aware of postpartum depression) _____

_____

Places you can go with your infant when you need
to get out of the house (parks, another new mom's house) _____

_____

_____

_____

*See Nurturing Yourself
During Pregnancy; the
Postpartum sections; and
Isn't Self-Nurturing
Impossible with Infants
and Toddlers? for help
coming up with ideas.*

Things you plan to do to nurture yourself
in the first few days after the baby is born (be specific). _____

_____

_____

In addition, collect and put into a folder with your list:

• Collection of take-out menus, especially places that deliver;

• Phone number of a late-night or all-night pharmacy, especially one
  that delivers;

• If you don't have a car, phone numbers of cab services or a neighbor with a car;

• Emergency numbers posted by the phone, including your doctor
  and partner or best friend's work number.

General Postpartum Preparedness Notes

If at all possible, hire someone to do your heavy cleaning. Every two
weeks for fourteen weeks is perfect. (No, perfect is every day forever!
Every two weeks for a limited amount of time is realistic.)

Simplify the running of your home as much as possible. Even water-
ing plants can feel impossible in the first few months. Look around at
what takes extra time and energy. Can you put away knickknacks?
Loan plants to a friend? Store anything you feel compulsively driven to
straighten or clean?

If you have a partner who will be home with you, the crunch may
come when your mate goes back to work. All your helpers may leave
around the same time and colic may descend just when your exhaustion is hitting a peak. Consider staggering your help to cover this time
by having less help the first week and more the third; by hiring someone to help a few hours a day in the first two weeks after your partner
returns to work; by running away and joining the circus (sorry, I was
listening to my screaming baby when I wrote that); and by alerting
friends and family that the first two weeks may be a grace period and

you will really need their love and hands afterward. You might tell them, "Don't disappear when you think we want privacy." You'll want privacy in the first few days and weeks. Later, it can become isolation.

Prepare Emotional Support

Your need for attention and an understanding ear does not disappear when the baby appears. It increases dramatically. But people tend to forget the mother and focus on the baby, which, while it makes you proud, can also make you feel forgotten, resentful, and lonely. Organize emotional support now:

Ask family and friends, especially ones who live far away, to send you "support cards," notes or postcards telling you everything will be okay and that you are doing a great job. Stress that they don't have to be elaborate; you just need to know you still count.

Invite a friend or two to call every few days and ask about you, not the baby. It is especially wonderful to have at least one friend who can listen to you moan about the dark side of becoming a mom without making you feel bizarre or ungrateful.

If you are going back to work, have a working mom who has gone before ready to comfort you without your having to ask. Explain to your supporter your fears and give that person the date when you will be returning.

Gifts for the mom are the best. I got a gooey chocolate cake from my editor, a plant from best buddy Barbra, and flowers from several wonderful friends. Yes, it would be indescribably rude to ask for gifts. So hint broadly to someone who won't be offended.

Resources:

Breast-Feeding National Network / Medela. Phone 800-835-5968. A twenty-four-hour recorded telephone service provided by breast pump manufacturer Medela. Punch in your ZIP code to find the closest place to rent a Medela pump and also the name and numbers of local lactation consultants or visit http://www.medela.com.

Canadian Lactation Consultant Association, 852 Knottwood Road South, Edmonton, Alberta T6K 3C3, Canada. Phone 403-462-1848. Call for a referral for your area. Serves all of Canada with over 200 members.

International Lactation Consultants' Association, 1500 Sunday Drive, Suite 102, Raleigh, NC, 27607. Phone 919-861-5577 for a referral to a lactation consultant or other support person in your locale. Visit http://www.ilca.org

La Leche League International. Phone 800-LA-LECHE (9 A.M. to 3 P.M. Eastern Time) or 847-519-7730 for the name of your local La Leche League leader or for a catalog of books, pamphlets, and breast pumps. Can also refer you to La Leche help in other countries. Best bet is http://www.lalecheleague.org

National Association of Postpartum Care Services. Supplies a list of postpartum care services or doulas in your area. Visit http://www.napcs.org or call 800-453-6852.

Operating Instructions: A Journal of My Son's First Year, by Anne Lamott (Ballantine Books, 1994). The hilarious, touching diary of a single mother's first year.

The Complete Book of Breastfeeding, by Marrin Eiger and Sally Olds (New York: Workman, 1999). Another good choice.

The New Mom's Companion: Care for Yourself While You Care for Your Newborn, by Debra Gilbert Rosenberg and Mary Sue Miller (Source Books, 2003). Written for any new mother with questions about mothering.

The Nursing Woman's Companion, by Kathleen Hughes, R.N., M.S. (National Book Network, 1999). An excellent breast-feeding book. Highly recommended.

Websites:

Hip Mama
http://www.hipmama.com

Mom's Companion
http://www.momscompanion.com

Myria
http://www.Myria.com

A Baby and Mother
Blessing Journey

When to Do It:

- Four to six weeks before your due date is ideal.

- If you are feeling alone, without the tradition or support of other women to draw on.

- If you wish you could have a whole group of your friends with you during the birth.

- When you want to draw on the wisdom and power of women throughout time.

What Is It?

We all have fears about giving birth. We know billions of women have come before us, triumphantly crossing the threshold of birthgiving to become mothers, but how can we keep that thought with us, especially during labor? We know many people love us and wish us well, but how can we wrap that love around us, remember it? Draw on it by using the power of ritual and the support of a group of women you choose.

This ritual journey is designed to provide you with a relaxing, imaginative, loving experience and to give you courage during labor and into the early months of being a mother. You might like this ritual to be a complete surprise. If so, choose a trusted friend or two to lead the ceremony, give them this book, and read no farther than What to Do. If you would like to be involved in the planning, enlist your trusted

You'll Need:

Magical music that is particularly special to you, that you could also listen to during birth.

A list of supportive women.

A private space, indoors or outdoors, large enough for your group to sit in a circle.

Note: Additional items needed, but I've listed these under What to Do so that if you want this to be a surprise, you won't know all the details.

friends anyway. You cannot lead the ritual; you must relax and experience it. With your friend(s), draw up a list of women whom you would like to participate.

If it feels truly impossible to gather a group, record the meditation part of the ceremony, create a sacred space for yourself, and modify the ceremony to do alone. You can also do this as part of or in place of a more traditional baby shower.

What to Do: Stop Reading Here if You Want This to Be a Surprise

This ritual was originally created with Randi Ragan for Kristina Coggins and our women's spirituality group.

Prepare

Preparing entails sending out invitations, gathering the materials needed, and preparing the space to be quiet and comfortable. Read through the ceremony, making the ritual your own. Past additions have included reading a poem about birth; the pregnant woman reading a letter she has written to her unborn child; reading a pledge to the unborn child; and each woman talking about her experience of birth, including birthing creative projects.

The invitations you send can give some sense of what is going to happen and what people need to bring. A sample invitation:

> You are invited to participate in a baby blessing ceremony, hosted by Jennifer and Randi, for Kristina. This ceremony will include singing, meditation, offering Kristina our support, and gifts for her unborn child. The ceremony is relaxing and requires your interaction. We hope you can make it! (Please direct questions to us. Kristina knows nothing!)
>
> Please bring a symbolic gift that represents a quality or wish you would like to bestow on the baby. For example, you might bring a feather you find to represent the gift of a spiritual life. Or a small mirror to represent the gift of being truthful with oneself.

The idea is not to spend money, but to represent an intangible wish. Please bring a pillow or beach chair to sit on, and a candle.

It is a good idea to have the group assemble fifteen to thirty minutes or so before the pregnant woman is present, so that you can go over what everyone is going to say and do.

In addition to what the women bring, you will need to gather:

• Several pillows and two comfy blankets

• A hairbrush

• A drum or rattle

• The relaxing music that has been chosen

• A bowl of water with herbs in it and a washcloth

• A song of your choice printed on index cards for each person

See Resources for songs.

Prepare the space by lighting candles, burning sage, or diffusing scented oils. Play relaxing music. The best design for this ceremony is to have the women form a circle around the pregnant woman, who sits, and eventually lies down, in the center of the circle. Place the candles the participants bring in a semicircle near where her head will eventually lie.

Beginning the Ceremony

When the participants arrive, have them sit in a circle, bringing their gifts, their candles, and their pillows with them. Walk the women through the ritual, indicating where they will participate and how you will cue them. These participatory spots are marked by asterisks and are:

• Singing the song. The song is sung over and over again, until you give a cue for everyone to stop.

• Bathing the honored woman. One at a time, each woman will bathe the face and hands of the pregnant friend while repeating a line of reassurance. (Examples are given, or make up your own.)

- Laying hands on the pregnant woman. Each woman lays her hands on the forehead, shoulders, belly, knees, or feet of the pregnant woman and imagines sending healing, strengthening, empowering energy into her.

In addition, one woman needs to drum or rattle when you indicate for her to do so.

When the pregnant woman arrives, start the music and ask her to take her place in the middle of the circle.

The Journey

"We are here today to honor the wondrous event, the incredible transformation, that our friend _____ is in the process of creating. Let's begin by everyone closing her eyes and taking a few deep breaths. (Pause.) Coming into your center, allowing yourself to be calm. There is no place else to be but here, nothing else to be doing but honoring our friend. (Pause; remember to breathe and relax yourself too.) Imagine a circle of light, any color you choose, encircling the group. (Pause.) Now, imagine all the colors intertwining and encircling us in a gorgeous, protective rainbow. (Pause.)

"To help _____ remember that she deserves self-nurturing and attention, especially after the baby is born, we will each take turns brushing her hair. _____, allow yourself to relax and take in the attention.

"Is there anything you would like to share with us about your pregnancy or your feelings about birth? Specifically, how can we help you in the coming months? (This is a chance for the honored woman to read a letter to her unborn child, perhaps part of the journal she might have been keeping, and to ask for specific help for the coming months.)

"Going around the circle, let us each pledge one act of support for after the birth, something specific we can do.

"Now it is time for the meditation, for the journey to meet your ancestors. _____, lie down and close your eyes. (Help her get
comfortable and make sure she is warm enough.)

"This is a journey into the imagination for all of us. Together, we will
create the energy necessary to take _____ back into the
ancient mysteries. Let us all take a moment, again, to close our eyes
and sink down, down into our centers, as we are all about to start on
a remarkable, powerful journey. (Pause; relax and feel the energy of
the room. If it feels too tense or scattered, turn up the volume of the
music and keep encouraging everyone to breath for two or three
minutes.)

"_____, breathing in, breathing out, following your
breath deep within you, settling into your core of inner wisdom. You
are perfectly safe within our circle of light, within this circle of women
who love, respect, and want to nurture you. Allow the floor to fully
support you. Allow any tension to flow out of your body. You don't
need to do anything, you don't need to control this, just let go. Open
up and receive. (Speak slowly. Pause often. Sense how relaxed she is
and encourage her to let go more if necessary.)

"Traveling back through time and space, following your breath back,
back to a time when the mystery and power of birth was revered.
(Take your time.)

"When you are ready, you find yourself standing at the mouth of a
cave, with a torch in your hand. Somehow, you know it is the cave
that the women in your tribe use for all the mysteries of being a
women: first menstruation, preparing for birth, menopause. (Describe
what the opening of the cave looks like to you. Let your imagination
speak.) Take a moment to take this in, let it become real to you.
(Pause.)

"If you are willing and want to, taking your torch with you, climb into
the cave. You have to crawl into a damp and narrow space as you
enter. As you do, the memory of coming here for your first-blood ritual returns to you. You remember being lead here by your mother,
your sister, your aunt, and taught the power of being a woman. It feels

utterly safe and familiar, yet exciting, as you continue deeper into the cave. (Continue to guide your friend into the cave, explaining as you go what it looks like. You might describe cave paintings you see on the walls, gems gleaming in the torchlight, whatever feels right.)

"Dimly, you begin to hear the sound of chanting and drumming.* (Indicate to the group to begin singing and drumming softly.) You walk toward the sound. (Pause; let the song go for several rounds.)

"In time, you find yourself emerging into a large cavern, lit by many torches. The cavern is filled with the women who have come before you. (Describe women your friend might like to see: her mother, grandmother, aunts, the women present, native women of the land you live on, ancestors unknown but imagined. Tailor the description to her life history.) These women welcome you with their song. They beckon to you. The wisdom, the power, the beauty in this room nourishes you, astonishes you, moves you, sending energy and strength throughout your body. (Pause.)

"These women are all here tonight to honor and bless you, to help you prepare for your birth. Tenderly, they bathe you with consecrated herbal water, a gift from the Earth.* (Here each woman bathes the hands and face of the pregnant woman while repeating an affirmation. Some possible affirmations:

> There goes all fear you hold about giving birth. The birth will be perfect.
>
> There goes all fear you hold about healing. You will heal beautifully.
>
> There goes all fear you hold about not being a good mother. You will be enough.
>
> There goes all fear of never being creative again. You can have a life of your own.
>
> There goes the deepest, most private fears you have about giving birth. You will be enough.)

*In unison, repeat firmly: "You will be enough. You are strong enough.

"The light from the wisdom and experience of these women streams out of their hands to bless you.* (Here each woman takes turns laying her hands on the pregnant woman, silently imagining healing, loving energy streaming from her hands into the honored woman's body. Take lots of time here.)

"The power of all women is with you. (Here is the place to add your own touch: What special help or blessing does your friend need? What elements of her own spiritual beliefs could be incorporated now? Past additions have included reading a prayer, anointing the pregnant woman with cornmeal, talking about a past miscarriage, and a group massage.)

"You know the energy and blessing your friends have given you will protect you, will nourish you, through the coming months, through the birth. You know that you only have to remember this, and you will find the strength, the honesty, the courage you need.* (Indicate for the women to start singing the song softly again.) Make any farewells you wish, and when you are ready, you take your torch and, knowing the wisdom, the strength, the power, and the conviction are always with you, you walk back out. (Describe a little bit of what she saw on the journey into the cave but, obviously, in reverse order.) Coming back up, slowly, remembering the blessings, bringing the energy, knowing it is always available to you.

"When you are ready, come back to this room (name the town or person's house you are in), back to the circle, ready for our gifts and blessings for your baby."

The Gifts

Share your gifts now, remembering to tell her what qualities each one represents.

Ending

You might want to discuss the ending with the group beforehand. You might sit silently for a few moments, then say thank-you to everyone;

sing another song someone knows; lead everyone in a silent prayer; read a poem or quote about birth; put on rhythmic music, dancing together and letting go of the often intense energy this ritual raises.

It is always wonderful to close with a potluck feast. You could segue into a more traditional party at this point, with men and other women joining you.

Above all, take your time, nourish your spirit, and have fun!

Resources:

Sacred Ceremony: How to Create Ceremonies for Healing, Transitions, and Cele-brations, by Steven D. Farmer (Hay House, 2002). Ideas on how to create your own ceremonies to consecrate the critical events and passages of life – like having a baby.

The Book of New Family Traditions: How to Create Great Rituals for Holidays & Everydays, by Meg Cox (Running Press, 2003). A fantastic manual—inspired.

The Joy of Family Rituals: Recipes for Everyday Living, by Barbara Biziou (St. Martin's Press, 2000). Recipes you can adapt to create your own blessing way, baby shower or naming day.

Welcoming Ways: Creating Your Baby's Welcome Ceremony With the Wisdom of World Traditions (Cedco Publishing, 2000). Available through http://www.Ambledance.com

Websites:

Lady Slipper
http://www.ladyslipper.org—approximately 15,000 (and growing!) current and past artists and titles

Baby Names
http://www.babycenter.com/babyname

Blessing Work
http://www.theblessingworks.com

Postbirth Nourishment

Surviving and Thriving

When to Do It:

- From birth on. *Every day.*

- Whenever the dear, precious angel (or sometimes #&$@#) is asleep.

- When you haven't slept in three months.

What Is It?

There will be few times in your life when taking care of yourself will be more important than it will be for the next year.

There will be no time in your life when taking care of yourself will be more difficult.

The importance of being good to yourself, arranging for others to be good to you, and allowing yourself to accept their help must not be underestimated. In the first weeks, your life can literally depend on it; you are in danger of postpartum hemorrhage for two weeks after birth, and doing too much too soon dramatically increases your chances of hemorrhage. Your sanity can hinge on it; a number of pioneers working in the field of postpartum depression believe the lack of nurturing women receive postpartum is directly linked to the severity and length and sometimes even the onset of depression. Your relationship with your baby can be affected: while most people agree the fixation on bonding is overdone, if you have twins, a premature or ill baby, or a "high need" or "fussy" baby like I did and you aren't getting any

You'll Need:

People to cuddle the baby, bring you appetizing meals, and send you loving cards and thoughtful gifts.

Portable, prepared comforts such as lilac soap, graham crackers, a porch swing, or a recording of Gregorian chants.

A comfortable breast-feeding station.

The belief that to nurture your child, you must nurture yourself.

breaks, you are going to momentarily hate that baby. That will make you feel the most intense guilt and self-loathing imaginable. How can you have any negative feelings about this perfect, innocent being? Your perception of yourself as a mother might be affected; not enough sleep makes anyone feel incompetent and unlovable. I was convinced my daughter loved my husband more than me when she was only one month old! And as the first year of motherhood unfolds, you will certainly discover that if you don't pay scrupulous attention to your needs, you will get sick, exhausted, and utterly depleted very quickly. And you can't recover easily, because you have an infant to take care of. Don't start this vicious cycle!

But you may ignore this message and deny yourself even the most basic self-nurturing. Why? Because you are so enthralled with this miniature human in your arms, because you are overwhelmed by the amount of work it takes to care for this creature, because all the attention is centered on the baby, because you are pummeled by feelings of inadequacy, guilt, and perfectionism, or because it is simply easier and more familiar to deny yourself. *Almost every woman finds it easier to ignore her own needs than to take care of herself.* My hope it to convince you, cajole you, compel you to care for yourself. By doing so you can help to prevent illness, depression, resentment, and the setting up or deepening of a debilitating pattern for your life as a mother: Mom comes last, Mom doesn't matter, and, finally, Mom incinerates.

Let's deal with the physical survival issues and then in the next section talk about the perplexing and sometimes frightening emotional changes you may be experiencing.

What to Do:

The First Few Weeks

See How to Gracefully Ask for and Accept Support; and Preparing for Postpartum.

Rest, snooze, kick back, hibernate, and relax as much as you can for two weeks. Yes, *two* weeks. There will be dozens of reasons why you should, must, can, ought to resume your life after a few days. *Resist.* You may feel unable to ask others to help you. Open up and accept help, or you may face burnout and exhaustion. You might feel housebound and restless. Turn that around. Recall all the busy, exhausted times in your life when you would have killed for two weeks at home. *Stay put.* You may be bursting with energy and want to show your beautiful baby off. He or she will be just as precious in two weeks. It is much better for both of you to *lie low.* Birth is not an illness, and you don't have to stay in bed (although that is a truly lovely idea), but it is amazingly easy to exhaust, overwhelm, and depress yourself. You really want to avoid that.

Sitz baths are very effective for sore bottoms. Take one a day for at least three days, especially if you had a vaginal delivery.

See Appendix: Herbs, Oils, and Other Natural Comforters for sitz bath recipes and how-to.

Of course, you've arranged for someone to feed you and your family nutritious and delicious meals. You will be ravenous. Enjoy it. *Do not for one moment worry about losing weight.* That subject is off-limits. As one friend says, "Don't go there." In other words, keep your mind out of that familiar dungeon of body obsession. If necessary, cover the mirrors in your bedroom and bathroom. At all costs, avoid the scale! Remind yourself that you just gave birth. Your body carried a baby and worked with that baby to bring it into the world; celebrate your flesh (or at least, don't abuse it).

Put a sign on your door that says something like, "We are the proud parents of Sam, 7 pounds, 9 ounces. We are *so* glad you've come by for a visit. Our doctor/midwife requested that in order for us to rest and get to know our baby, everyone limit their visits to fifteen minutes. We so want to share our new baby with you, and short visits are a good compromise." The Santa Barbara Midwives add to their sign, "Before you leave, it would be helpful if you lent a hand. Quietly wash up the dirty dishes or take the laundry home or water the plants or do any other nice thing you feel inclined to do!" (How can you ask Aunt Bell who drove all the way from Tulsa to stay only fifteen minutes? The best advice is keep her from coming in the first place. Or allow her thirty minutes and then retire to the bedroom "to nurse.")

Record a new greeting on your answering machine. Note your baby's name, birthdate, weight, and length, along with a gentle warning that you won't be returning phone calls promptly. If you have asked someone to coordinate helpers or field questions, put that person's name and phone number on your machine and instruct callers to get in touch with him or her.

Arrange to receive a massage from a friend, or hire someone to come to your house. One woman I interviewed had a tough labor, which ended in a C-section. She had a masseuse give her a full-body massage two days after she returned home and felt "it began the healing process."

Write your labor and birth story. Every woman's birthgiving is worthy of celebration. It might help to write your story as if you were telling it to your newborn. You may find yourself weeping, swearing, cringing, or smiling. That's part of the process. Do this before you forget. Verbalize your story too. Recounting the drama to as many sympathetic listeners as possible helps make the whole astounding endurance test and the baby in your arms more real. If you had a rough time, talking can ease the horror. Get together a group of friends to listen to your story (at a friend's house, not yours, because you do not want to be entertaining) several weeks after the birth for the healing ritual of being listened to.

See I Am a Body Without
a Brain: Postpartum
for more.

Celebrate the spiritual dimension of this time. Meditate on your newborn's feet while he or she eats (baby feet are the essence of God). Don't think, just marvel and breathe. Note your dreams; the interruption of your sleep cycle makes them easier to remember. Don't do anything with your dreams, simply reflect on one when you wake up to feed the baby. Sit outside and feel the wind on your skin, the earth under your feet. Step back for one minute once or twice a day to be astonished at the wonder of a new life and your emergence as a mother.

Breast-feeding and bottle-feeding can be hard on your back. Try to stretch a little each day. If you own a workout video, do just the stretching portion. Concentrate on lowering your shoulders, relaxing your jaw, and being aware of your posture while feeding and cradling your baby.

Remember to take your vitamins, especially extra calcium. It is just as important now as when you were pregnant.

Night sweats and hot flashes are all too common for the first month or longer. Scented powder or alcohol splashes help keep you from smelling like a longshoreman. There can also be an unpleasant odor caused by your bleeding. Using a spritz bottle to rinse your genitals every time you pee and changing your pad each time helps. So do multiple showers. Rubbing scented lotion on the insides of your thighs can disguise the odor.

From every mom I interviewed: *sleep when the baby sleeps.* Before baby arrives, this sounds easy and sensible. But you may be high and not want to sleep. Or after a few days of sleeping when the baby sleeps, you may crave a little adult company. You may be getting lots of phone calls and visitors. It is so easy (and almost inevitable) to get caught up in the joy and suddenly find you are worn out. Minimize this by only doing half of what you normally would. If you are breast-feeding, sleeping when the baby sleeps may mean you only have a half-hour to two-hour slot. If you say to yourself after he drops off, "I'll just start a load of laundry" and that becomes "I'll just address a few birth announcements," then suddenly your baby is awake and ready to eat again. For at least the first month, when the baby is asleep, focus on yourself and rest. If that means sleep (which it often does), *sleep first.* If you don't want to or can't sleep, loll in bed and read something that transports you. Or meditate for ten minutes. Do whatever restores and centers you. If you have other children to take care of, it is imperative you focus on yourself and rest for at least the first two weeks, and if that is utterly impossible, then at least two of your baby's sleep periods out of the day and early evening must be yours.

See Preparing for Postpartum.

If you truly can't stand a mess, take five minutes (no more!) to straighten your bedroom, then shut the door and loaf around. Remind yourself that no one ever died of a dirty bathroom. (Maybe somebody slipped on a greasy floor, your critical voice mutters. Tell that voice to take a hike; you just gave birth!) Remind yourself you wouldn't expect anyone else recovering from a major physical endurance test (or surgery if you had a cesarean) to dust every book in the house or even to wash the sheets every week.

The best advice for the first two weeks? *Do half of what you think you are capable of.* Take it slower and easier than you feel you need to. Cut out everything that isn't vital to your baby's and your health and mental well-being. This time will never come again. Focus on yourself and your baby, and forget about unreturned phone calls, in-laws, and work.

Postpartum Comforts

The challenge of surviving the next few months without imbibing excessive amounts of chocolate, wine, and daytime TV talk shows depends on rest, support, and a handy bag of comforts. This may be one of the most emotionally and physically draining experiences of your life. Or it may not be; it depends on your labor, your baby, your support system, and a host of individual and cultural factors. Either way, you will be getting less sleep and carrying more responsibility than ever before. Comfort is required! Try any of these suggestions that appeal to you:

Escape for a one- to two-hour outing to your "old life." I yearned to wander around my favorite bookstore. Corey craved her early morning walk on the beach. Janet wanted to have lunch with colleagues from work and not talk about feeding schedules and infant stimulation. Mary simply wanted to follow her old morning routine of making tea a certain way. Do any activity that anchors you in familiar territory, even for a few minutes.

Attend a postpartum exercise class; they often offer child care. When it seems impossible to leave the house with a screaming baby, this is one place you can go and get sympathy instead of irked stares. The exercise makes you feel less despairing about your body, but, best of all, you get to see and talk to other exhausted mothers. (Even if you aren't a joiner and you don't need to make any new friends, go anyway. The community will do you good.)

Sometimes talking to other mothers is depressing because they seem to have all the answers or they have no conception of the emotional rigors of colic, prematurity, sibling rivalry, an unsupportive mate, or whatever you are enduring. Listen politely, then walk away and talk to yourself in your evil twin voice: "My baby doesn't sleep because she is brilliant. That baby of hers is headed for a lifetime career at McDonald's. Did you notice how beady his eyes are?" (Yes, sisterhood is great, but being wicked in the privacy of your own mind is sometimes imperative.)

Have your partner take a night feeding once a week. If your mate complains about needing to sleep because of a paltry excuse like work, have him or her take a weekend feeding. If you are breastfeeding, express milk. Sleep away from baby and mate in another room or in the yard in a tent (if you are laughing, you obviously aren't sleep deprived yet). If you are a single mom, have a friend in to help or, if possible, hire a night nanny. Four to eight hours of uninterrupted sleep is the absolute best comfort of all.

Read what other mothers have gone through. Pick up *Operating Instructions* by Anne Lamott, *Mothers Talking* by Frances Wells Burck, *Mother Zone* by Marni Jackson, or *The Wish, The Wait, The Wonder* compiled by Gail Perry Johnston.

Sometimes, returning to old and not-so-great ways of comforting yourself is all that will get you through the day or night. Eating is the first choice of mothers everywhere, and for good reasons. During pregnancy, you may have allowed yourself to eat without restraint, perhaps for the first time in your adult life. It can be very hard to stop. Nursing brings with it a voracious appetite. Food provides an effective buffer, taking the edge off the intense emotions that may be battering you. Food is soothing; it is perhaps one of the few pleasures available to you in the isolation of caring for a newborn, and it can serve as emotional sustenance to keep you going when you have nothing left to give. My advice? Don't consider the D word (dieting) until you have a little control and confidence in your life, which could be as long as a year to eighteen months. If you are nursing, dieting is *not* recommended, as it can affect your milk supply. Try to eat healthily, but avoid putting additional pressure on yourself. If you have a history of food disorders, consider discussing this with a counselor. Give yourself a break: this is probably going to be one of the most stressful times of your life. You will have plenty of time to get back into shape when you are getting more sleep. Don't waste precious energy beating yourself up.

When you are changing diapers, repeat a few affirmations aloud to yourself and your baby. "I am the best mother for my child" is my favorite, especially when I'm feeling totally inadequate. "I am growing every day as a mother and a person." "When I nurture myself, I nurture my baby." "All is well." Don't tune out the negative, critical voice that may pipe up. Listen politely but with detachment. Comprehend how willing you may be to beat yourself up. Then keep on doing your best.

When you attend your last health care appointment, it is not unusual to feel sad or at a loss. Many women grieve the specialness of pregnancy and how much easier it is to take care of the baby when it is inside of you! Take a few moments to mark this passage. Sip some tea in a sidewalk cafe and write in your journal about how you feel. If child care is impossible, go for a walk with your baby on your chest and say good-bye to being pregnant.

Breast-Feeding Comfort

If you choose to breast-feed, *keep trying*. Many, many women reported the important of persistence. Keep trying; it is worth it; it *does,* in most cases, get much easier. It is worth it not only for your child's health but because it can be a soul-nurturing, time-saving, and money-saving experience for you.

Remember that breast-feeding is a *learned* art. It takes time and training to get it right. It can take a month or two. Do not despair. You are not an evolutionary reject. It is natural to take it personally when your child refuses or struggles with your breast. Take a break away from your baby for a few minutes and talk to yourself in your most reassuring, calming voice: "There is nothing wrong with me. I am a good mother. The baby doesn't hate me." Next, get help (see below). Finally, find another mom who has had trouble and commiserate over a glass of wine or a brownie fudge sundae.

The best possible advice for breast-feeding moms: if you experience *any* difficulties, call a lactation consultant *immediately*. (Many hospitals have them on staff.) If you don't know of one and have a crisis in the middle of the night, try your midwife or a nurse in the hospital where you gave birth. Don't suffer through difficulties alone. So often simply learning how to position your infant will change your whole world.

POSTBIRTH
NOURISHMENT

See Preparing for Postpartum: Preparing to Breast-Feed for help locating a lactation consultant.

The average mom spends one thousand hours breast-feeding her baby. Set up a breast-feeding station with a very comfortable chair that allows your feet to touch the floor (or use a footstool) and offers great back support. (A glider rocker is a worthwhile investment.) A neck pillow (U-shaped) to support the baby and give your arm a rest is very helpful. The U curves around your waist and under your arms. For extra comfort (although this is a bit involved) add two small tables (TV trays work perfectly) on either side of your chair. On one table, put a phone, a pitcher of water and a glass (or a sports bottle with a flexible straw), TV remote control, spit-up cloth, books and magazines, snacks that can be eaten with one hand, fingernail clippers for baby (nursing is a good time to trim), and lip balm for Mom. When you sit down to nurse on one side, switch your water and any other necessary goodies to the table on the side of your free hand. In the beginning, you might not have a free hand, but in time you will. (This chair situation is most helpful in the first few weeks. Of course, you can nurse anywhere. Just be sure to have fluids nearby and to have good back support.)

Breast-feeding time is prime self-nurturing time. Be in the moment of stillness while you gaze at your baby's exquisite face and marvel at the fact he or she is thriving on what your body produces. Read a great novel or poetry aloud or listen to a book on tape (your library probably has many titles or see if your video store rents audios). Watch an old movie (I hate TV, but cable can be a worthwhile investment for these first few months, or rent a favorite film and watch in snippets while nursing). Meditate by focusing on the sound of your baby's sucking. Listen to a guided imagery tape, a late-night talk radio show, or Native American flute music (on headphones late at night). Keep a tape recorder at hand, let your mind wander, and record your ideas. Unwind while you enjoy the hormonal rush.

POSTBIRTH
NOURISHMENT

*See Receiving the
Nurturing You Need from
Your Partner Postpartum
(and Giving a Little Too):
Gatekeeping.*

Include your partner in breast-feeding. Feed the baby lying on your side in bed between you and your partner. If your baby enjoys it, your mate can massage his legs, stroke her back, or, better yet, rub your feet and tickle your back! Your mate can burp the baby, change diapers before or afterward, soothe the baby, and put her down. Just because you are breast-feeding does not mean the baby is "your" responsibility.

You will sometimes wish you could take off your boob and hand it to someone else to nurse your baby. You may feel "attached at the tit," as Mimi, mother of Molly, delicately put it. Gratification and enjoyment may be mixed with feeling trapped. Practice surrender. Curse. If you have a partner, roll over and say, "You nurse her this time" (humor helps). Pump a bottle so you can go to a movie or take a nap and skip a feeding.

Comfort When You Can't Breast-Feed

The inability to breast-feed, or having problems with it, can be truly devastating. The message today is that you are a terrible mother if you don't breast-feed. You may feel like your body failed you. You may wonder if you will "bond" sufficiently with your child. If your pediatrician recommends supplementing with formula, that too can feel like an indictment of your womanhood. Many women and babies have difficulties breast-feeding. This is not abnormal. Women who have had breast cancer or lumpectomies will face special challenges.

No matter what you think or feel now, please know *your child will not be scarred for life if you cannot breast-feed.* However, if you wish to breast-feed and aren't getting the support you need or are in pain, please get competent help before you quit.

While breast-feeding is wonderful for your baby, nobody talks about the impact it can have on you as a mother—how all-consuming, how emotionally difficult, how claustrophobic it can feel. You may experience:

- Confusing feelings of dependency during breast-feeding. Emotions or memories you have defended yourself against for years can surface around feeding your baby.

- Anger if nursing doesn't go perfectly or if your baby has trouble latching on. You can feel rejected by a sleepy baby or one who has a hard time sucking. The anger, resentment, or frustration you may feel at an infant who can't or won't nurse, coupled with the incredible physical and emotional changes you are going through postbirth, can leave you feeling like the bottom of a dirty birdcage.

- Receiving inaccurate instruction in learning to nurse. Breast-feeding classes can make it seem simple, rarely discussing the idiosyncratic problems you may run into (no one told me it was okay if Lillian only took one breast at a feeding and would only nurse on the left side for the first six weeks).

- Not having enough time. If you have other children, the extra time it takes to breast-feed can be hard to juggle and can make your toddler or older child jealous.

- The hassles of going back to work. This is a challenge for almost every working woman. Few workplaces are supportive of the time and space needed to pump. It can be very difficult to get your milk to let down standing in a bathroom. You'll be working and feel your breasts tingling and think, "Oh no, time to pump again. But I just got into my work." Try doing this in the middle of a meeting: "Excuse me, I have to go pump my breasts" might not go over well.

- Shyness at nursing in public and feeling trapped at home because of it. If you are suffering from isolation or postpartum depression, this can be the last straw in your ability to cope.

- Sexual arousal. This is completely normal, although it can be very disconcerting, especially if you have been sexually abused or feel ambivalent about yourself as a sexual being.

- An unsupportive or jealous partner. Your mate may think breast-feeding is weird or for "hippies." Or he or she may want you to be available for travel or to resume your life with as little change as possible.

- An overwhelming need to see yourself as separate and to regain your sense of self. Breast-feeding intensifies and prolongs the feeling of being one with your infant, which can psychologically be very overwhelming.

Whatever the reasons, if Mom doesn't do it perfectly, Mom is made to feel she failed her baby. Breast-feeding is rarely easy, and like all of parenting it can't be totally controlled by you. If you have tried to breast-feed and been unable to, you may feel dreadful. You may feel no one understands how important this was to you. *I do and so do many other women.* This experience has the power to plant seeds of self-doubt about yourself as a mother and to undermine your confidence in other areas too. ("I couldn't even breast-fed. Maybe I can't do anything right for my baby. Maybe my baby doesn't love me.") If anyone (from your mother to a nurse in the hospital) criticizes you for not breast-feeding, you will feel even more "deficient." Comfort yourself by:

- Finding another woman who has had problems and ask her how she felt and what helped her get through. Ask your health care provider, or ask close friends if they know anyone who chose not to or was unable to breast-feed.

*See Ambivalence:
Grieving the Changes.*

- Grieving if it feels appropriate to grieve. Don't downplay your feelings.

- Forgiving yourself for failing. Don't let this hang over you like a dark cloud. Forgive yourself and move on to avoid getting into the feeling of having to make it up to your child.

- Talking to your mate so that the subject of breast-feeding doesn't become an area of resentment between you. (It is oh so easy to project our anger onto our partners during this emotionally vulnerable time.) Although it seems impossible for a man to grasp how important it can be to breast-feed your baby, try to communicate your feelings. You may need to realize your mate cannot fully understand what you are going through. Try not to blame him.

- Knowing in your heart that no single act of loving parenting makes or breaks your child. *You have not ruined your child or compromised his or her health.*

Sleep

Keep repeating to yourself, "I will get through this. I did not make a mistake." Your body will adjust to less sleep. The hormones help.

It is easy to become obsessed with sleep. Counting how many hours you got last night. Querying other mothers on how much their babies sleep. "Embrace the differences," said Fredda, a single mother. "Stop wishing for how it was." Wishing for a six- to eight-hour block of sleep just makes you feel more deprived and resentful. Congratulate yourself on how well you are doing. Make naps your number one priority, if possible, even after you go back to work (nap at lunchtime). Avoid operating heavy machinery, especially piloting commercial aircraft.

However, do not ignore the power of sleep deprivation to wreck your life. Sleep deprivation has been known to cause irritability, paranoid thinking, hallucinations, and episodic rages. If your life is beginning to unravel, you need more sleep. Ask or hire someone to watch the baby and give him or her a bottle (you can pump if you are breast-feeding), thereby buying a four- to six-hour stretch of uninterrupted sleep. For a week, sleep when the baby sleeps, even if your house becomes filthy and your other child(ren) hate you. You must get rest! If you are back at work, you might need to take a day off to sleep. *The importance of sleep cannot be overemphasized.* Take it from someone whose baby was still waking up every two hours at six months: sleep is essential.

If getting back to sleep after waking to feed or soothe the bambino is hard, make a thermos of herbal tea. Steep 1 part chamomile, 1 part linden blossom, 1 part lavender, and 1 part valerian root tea for ten to twenty minutes, then keep by your bed. Try establishing a going-back-to-sleep ritual. Perhaps you read for fifteen minutes. Or pray. Or fold laundry. Or keep all lights low and talk only in baby sounds.

Recovering Emotionally from an Unplanned Cesarean Birth

(Many of these ideas are also helpful for recovering from a premature birth or bedrest.) The hardest part of recovering from a C-section, besides the gas, are the feelings of failure, anger, and betrayal: "Why did this have to happen to me?" You may have gotten the message (which most women do) that if you were a real woman, if you had practiced more Kegels, if you had chosen a different hospital, if you had labored at home longer, if you hadn't asked for pain meds so soon, you could have birthed vaginally. The what-ifs can eat you alive.

Everybody says to you, "You should be happy. You have a beautiful baby. That's all that matters." Hearing this doesn't help. It may make you feel guilty: "What's the matter with me? Why do I feel so bad about not having a vaginal delivery?" It may make you angry: "I don't care about the baby. I feel cheated. I (we) spent months preparing for a natural delivery, and that's what I wanted." This well wishing may make you feel misunderstood, isolated, and silly for not letting your cesarean go. But consider the reasons you may feel bad:

- "Natural" childbirth has become almost a moral imperative. If you ask for drugs, the implication is you are a bad person. It is also implied that if you can't cut the mustard by having a vaginal delivery, you are really a weak woman. This nasty attitude can subtly appear in your postbirth conversations with health care providers, friends, and other new moms who didn't have a C-section.

- An unplanned or emergency cesarean leaves you with little or no time to prepare. You might have been laboring in a softly lit room with just your mate or birth partner, when suddenly a dozen or more people are running around, poking you and the baby. You may have become very frightened, panicked, or felt out of control.

- You may not have believed a C-section could happen to you, especially if you planned a home birth or this is your second or third child.

- You may feel the child didn't come from you, that he or she was given or shown to you. Because of this, you may not feel as close to your baby as you expected. That alone can be devastating.

- You may find yourself blaming your birth partner, health care provider, or your new baby for your cesarean. That can make you feel horrible.

- Perhaps worst of all, you may feel physically mutilated, "ruined," or violated.

To begin the healing process, consider:

Your feelings don't have to make rational sense. When you add up major surgery, pain, the effects of drugs, failed expectations, and what can feel like a direct assault on your femininity, no wonder you may feel crazy, strange, full of rage, out of it, depressed, or inadequate. Don't add beating yourself up for having these feelings to the list.

Keep repeating to yourself, "Birth is a mystery. There are no guarantees." You are not God; you cannot control or predict what will happen.

If you can handle it, ask to have your baby room-in. Keep your baby close by you as much as possible. It can be immensely healing and reassuring to see that pink, old-man face and those infinitely wise eyes.

Nursing your baby can restore your trust in your body. The football hold makes it possible after a C-section. Have someone *experienced* show you how and support the baby until you get comfortable.

See Preparing for Postpartum: Preparing to Breast-Feed.

Ask for help. Accept pain medication if that feels okay to you. Do not exhaust yourself trying to do it all or trying to "make up" for having a C-section. There is nothing to make up for.

Find at least one other mother who has had a C-section. There are support groups available. Even if you have to drag yourself, try going to one meeting. Reach out to someone who has been through the same experience. (I know, it seems like my solution for everything, but support postbirth is so soothing and sanity promoting, it can't be overemphasized.)

Remember that any other person recovering from major surgery would not be required to take care of an utterly helpless newborn immediately afterward. Repeat that to yourself if you feel inadequate for not recovering faster or not doing more. You just gave birth!

If you feel you were treated impersonally or rudely or that procedures were inadequately explained to you, or if you are otherwise unhappy with your doctor, nurse, midwife, or any other medical professional, write that person a letter. Explain how you feel you were wronged. Be fair but honest and very specific. It can also help to write a letter to your baby, giving vent to your frustration, anger, or guilt. You might like to burn this one and bury the ashes with a bit of your baby's cord, to signify how both of you are growing into the future.

The joy you feel over having a baby will not lessen your physical pain, nor will it necessarily lessen your disappointments. That's okay.

Be aware that a cesarean can be bruising and disorienting for your mate or birth partner as well. Your partner may feel shame that he or she couldn't protect you from the surgery. A feeling of failure is common—that if the mate had only done what he or she was supposed to during labor, this wouldn't have happened. If your partner's mother had a cesarean, your cesarean may trigger primal feelings of helplessness and rage. *Talk about your feelings.* Don't hide from each other. Give yourselves time to heal. Wendy and her partner found taking an infant massage class together helped them bond with their baby and open up about their feelings.

Although you will worry if you haven't fallen in love with your baby yet, try to remember it can take weeks, even months. Chris and I began to enjoy parenting a little at six months and really fell in love at eight months. You aren't a monster. You are experiencing a normal, if traumatic, adjustment. Talk about it with someone who can understand.

Redefining Time

One of the most distressing things about becoming a mother is the way time changes. You lose control. Someone else is calling the shots. Before, you had to answer to the time requirements of your job, but you could still make choices. You could choose to quit, to take a day off, to switch projects because you were bored. With baby, choice becomes a memory. You cannot choose to take a day off; it must be arranged, planned for, negotiated (and if you are breast-feeding, you may spend two weeks pumping enough milk to leave and spend the time you are away pumping as well). You cannot choose not to care for the baby. You are called out of bed, interrupted in midsentence, made to leave the shower with soap in your hair.

In addition to losing control, the familiar measurements of time are banished. Clocks means nothing. For the first time in years, you may find yourself not wearing a watch (I had to call a friend to find out the date, and then there was the time I had to ask Chris what year it was). Your baby's demands for food, dry diapers, and attention regulate your day. With this dizzying feeling of losing choice and control comes the anxious feeling of never having enough time. Your baby goes to sleep for his or her nap. As soon as the eyes close, this giant, time-eating, anxiety-producing clock starts ticking in your belly. "Ten minutes is gone already and I haven't decided what to do. I've got to relax. What do I want to do with myself? He's going to wake up. I know he is going to wake up. I want to exercise, then shower, then nap. I'll never get to do all that. I should play it safe and get in the shower now." I would find myself dashing through whatever I needed to do as soon as Lillian napped or when it was Chris's time to care for her. After a few weeks, I felt like I was constantly in a panic. And while that calmed down as I adjusted to motherhood (and got more sleep), the very real presence of the Time Monster did not. Every moment had to be accounted for. Either I was trying to squeeze errands in between her naps or grab nap time while Grandmother baby-sat or exercise while Lillian played in the gym nursery or make love while she napped.

The sooner you can redefine time, the less frustrated and resentful you will be. To do this, you need to do two things. One, live in baby time. That means when you are with baby, you are with baby. The less you try to get accomplished and the more you live in the moment, the more enjoyable your life will be. Stop worrying about going back to work, making muffins for the mom's group, or how out of shape you are. Surrender your agenda for the moment. But you can't always be in baby time, or you will lose your sense of self and end up feeling smothered and irritable, plus you won't do simple things like eat. So you design a little cha-cha: a little baby time in which you don't try to get anything else done, except what is most pressing, like drink water, eat a sandwich, or pee, then a little adult time, in which you might have a conversation about something besides the color of poop, read a book that doesn't have pictures, or simply reclaim a tiny sense of your personal boundaries.

Second, when baby is otherwise occupied (which in the first few months can mean fifteen minutes to an hour if you're lucky or if your mate, mother, or a baby-sitter is present), you throw yourself into what most needs to be done. Grab the chunks of time you have, do what most needs to be done *in that moment,* and forget about the rest. Of course, what most needs to be done includes taking care of yourself. When you catch yourself panicking, "She's going to wake up from her nap before I'm done," or "I only have one more hour of child care and I have to get all this stuff done," stop. Take a deep breath and say to yourself, "There is enough time. I'm doing _____ _____ right now, and that is all that matters." When baby is no longer occupied, you must be willing to drop what you are doing and go back to being in baby time, releasing yourself from feeling you have failed to be productive or to relax or whatever.

Baby time also means not beating yourself up at the end of your day for not getting the house vacuumed or your home-based business started or networking phone calls to your office made. *Don't judge a good day by how much you used to get done.* Judge it by how much you could be wholeheartedly with your infant, how often you were able to surrender your agenda, how much you could be good to yourself and your children, how much you could learn today from a gas smile or an intense bout of screaming. Many days, just surviving is cause for a chorus of hallelujahs.

Baby time means trying to resist the temptation to do too much in one day. The only way baby time works is if you scale back! In the first few months, trying to exercise, make dinner, and go grocery shopping is probably too much for one day. Try for two of those things. If you are consistently trying to get too much done, if you can't relinquish your internal clock that pushes you to be on time or to have a schedule, you can't relax with your baby.

Don't get into the habit of putting work before self-nurturing. Self-nurturing must come first, at least some of the time, or it won't happen.

If or when you go back to work, switching back and forth between baby time and in-the-world time can be troublesome. Designing a transition ritual helps. Jamie changes into loose, comfy clothes, then nurses Ann while listening to classical music. Shana always leaves her work shoes outside the door and slips on house shoes. Lin leaves her briefcase in the car.

Remember, this period of time is amazingly brief. Once you are out of it, you may look back and have a hard time believing how quickly it went by. As one woman said, "Don't blink." Don't end up with regrets because you tried to force yourself always to live by linear time. See if you can enter into the timelessness of your baby's world. That alone will nurture you.

When Is My Life Supposed to Return to Normal?

Because the lochia (bleeding) stops and your uterus returns to its non-reproductive state by six weeks, it has become written in stone that six (maybe eight) weeks is the amount of time a woman, a baby, and a family are allowed to adjust. You better be back at work, back to your prepregnancy weight (or even a few pounds slimmer if you are breast-feeding because it burns so many extra calories), back to normal in all respects by this time. This is an arbitrary, ridiculous, and cruel demarcation. The amount of time it takes you to fold this sweet new spirit into your life is completely unique to you and your family. Forget competing to see who can fit into her jeans fastest or who is back to chauffeuring half the neighborhood. Curse the parent in the pediatrician's office whose baby started sleeping through the night at two weeks. Drop the friends (single) who make you feel weird because you don't want to take the baby out to dinner and the symphony. *Rebel against anyone who reinforces the idea that a mother today should be able to do everything.*

Whatever experience you are having, *you are not alone.* If you are having an easy time, great, enjoy it (but be careful when you flaunt it;

sleep-deprived people are dangerous creatures). If you feel like a cup of Jell-O (your thighs and your psyche), and your child cannot be put down for more than two minutes, you are not alone (at least I'm with you). One recent study found most women need from three months to eighteen months to recover fully from childbirth and raising an infant. Many women I spoke to said, "It took eighteen months before I felt like myself again." It helps to:

- Listen to what you need.

- Redefine normal.

- Ban *should* from your vocabulary.

Ignore the pressure of what is "normal" (a highly elusive concept anyway and usually defined by what others are saying you *should* do). Don't define this time by what you should be accomplishing. Listen to what your inner voice is saying your life needs to look like now. Sara, mother of Joe and an actress, found herself being pulled to go back to work six months postpartum. She felt conflicted about what to do. She spontaneously (with her son in a pack on her back) painted a picture one day. When she stepped back and studied it, she realized she had painted her answer: she needed to stay home for a full year. Although for many of us not working for a year is not an option, we do have other choices. Not attending your company picnic. Not returning phone calls. Pare your life to the minimum. Some people will not understand. The ones that do will stay in your life.

If you are feeling pulled, pressured, or abnormal, ask yourself, "What shoulds or harsh expectations are running my life right now?"

Keep telling yourself this time in your life is not permanent. You will sleep again. Borrow from the Twelve-Step programs—one day at a time. Above all, relax your own expectations and thumb your nose at others' expectations of you.

I need to say that again. *Relax your expectations and thumb your nose at others' expectations of you.* Besides isolation and lack of community, it is the unrealistic expectations we and others have for new moms that cause the greatest grief. (Lack of adequate maternity leave is another

huge one, and lack of respect for moms: I guess I could go on and on.)
Be sweet to your beautiful self. You are doing the best you can. And
your best is damn good.

Resources:

After the Baby's Birth, by Robin Lim (Berkeley: Celestial Arts, 1991). A nurturing, spiritual approach to postpartum. Includes physical exercises and
recipes.

Cesarean/Support, Education and Concern, 22 Forest Road, Framingham,
MA 01701. Phone 508-877-8266 for support recovering from a
C-section or help planning a VBAC.

Having a Cesarean Baby, by Richard Hausknecht, M.D., and Joan Rattner
Heilman (New York: Dutton, 1978). Thoughtful and complete but a
little dated.

Motherhood: What It Does to Your Mind, by Jane Price (London: Pandora,
1988). Excellent exploration of the psychological costs and adjustments.

Mothering the New Mother, by Sally Placksin (New York: Newmarket Press,
1994). Good resource for postpartum, especially for locating doulas
and postpartum depression clinics and assessing the troubling question
of going back to work.

Rebounding from Childbirth, by Lynn Madsen (Westport, CT: Bergin & Garvey,
1994). Wonderful book about healing from a traumatic birth.

The Premature Baby Book, by Helen Harrison (New York: St. Martin, 1984).
Comprehensive help.

The Year After Childbirth, by Sheila Kitzinger (New York: Scribners, 1994).
This book is inclusive (includes help for disabled women, survivors of
sexual abuse, single moms, lesbian moms, and mothers who are HIV-
positive), is written from a loving, feminist base, and offers information
about your well-being, not just your baby's.

Postbirth Nourishment

Surviving the Emotions

You'll Need:

Courage to reach out to others and to open your heart to the changes.

When to Do It:

- When your hormone levels plummet and you feel as beatific as the Madonna and as dumpy as Roseanne, trapped forever by leaking breasts, and in tears over a diaper commercial—all in the space of sixty seconds.

- When you are overcome with rage, anger, guilt, confusion, or regret.

- If you experience panic attacks, complete lack of interest in life or baby, obsessive thoughts of horrible things happening to you or your baby, a creeping feeling that everything isn't all right, and an inability to cope.

What Is It?

"Motherhood is like a storm, a seizure: It is like weather. Nights of high wind followed by calm mornings of dense fog or brilliant sunshine that gives way to tropical rain, or blinding snow," writes Laurie Colwin in her novel, *A Big Storm Knocked It Over.* No one can be prepared for the storm of emotional changes, revelations, fluctuations, and gyrations that occur in the days, weeks, months, and even up to a year following the birth of your child.

Having a baby was one of the most momentous emotional events of my life. Yet all I was prepared to feel was depressed. Some books I read suggested the entire emotional change consists of feeling weepy on day three! The range I felt and the changes I weathered were heart-boggling. You may never feel more flooded with love, more emotionally raw, more full of rage, more spiritually open, more numb, more exhausted, more lonely, or more needy. You may never feel less you, less ready, less able to cope, less competent.

More than anything, as new mothers we need permission to feel whatever comes up. Nothing is taboo, bad, weird, or creepy, nor are you ever alone in what you are feeling. It is the lack of permission to feel conflicted, inadequate, sad, angry, bored, or irritable as well as grateful, rapturous, tingling with life, and intoxicated with love that makes the postpartum period unnecessarily difficult and lonely.

Having a baby means giving birth to a new you. This disconcerting and momentous experience is pretty much ignored as well. You feel different yet the same. You may find yourself grieving for parts of your life that are gone forever (or at least for quite a while) and feel awkward with your new roles, likes, and dislikes. This vulnerable, itchy openness presents a fantastic opportunity for growth and change. As Deb, mother of Dakota, said, "I look at my postpartum distress as a blessing. By allowing myself to be vulnerable and look way down inside me, I was able to change in ways I needed to before I started to raise my baby." This is far from easy to do! New motherhood is such a bewildering and emotionally arduous time, but it is also exciting, ripe, and vivid.

Having a baby cracks your mind and heart wide open with joy and tenderness. Only rarely does anyone honestly, descriptively, and intimately talk or write about what else it can do—what I call the postpartum storm. This is a well-kept secret. We must come together and give a voice to our experience so that we can learn and grow from it, use it as the rich time it is, instead of numbing out because we have no context, no comparisons, and no one to support us. The emotional truth of having a baby is exhilarating and overwhelming; it connects you to your ancestors and confronts you with your childhood; it is miraculous and boring, peaceful and frightening, fulfilling and constricting. The emotional truth is, having a baby changes you, forever.

If you are afraid of how bad you are feeling or if you are experiencing panic attacks, or if at any time you contemplate hurting yourself or your infant, feel like you are drowning, or want nothing to do with your child, turn immediately to More Help at the end of this section.

What to Do:

A Word About Nomenclature

The only frank and in-depth discussion about postpartum adjustment that presently exists is under the label postpartum depression (also known as PPD; other names for increasing degrees of severity include maternity blues, postpartum stress syndrome, postpartum emotional difficulty, major postpartum depression, postpartum psychotic depression, and puerperal depression).

It is horrifying how many women have suffered and continue to suffer through postpartum depression, from the mildest form now called postpartum stress syndrome (which some researchers believe almost 100 percent of new moms suffer from) to the most severe, postpartum psychotic depression (exceedingly rare). It is critical to educate people about the reality and range of PPD and name the experience so women don't feel alone. But you may find the names limiting. Many women find the postpartum adjustment intense and disquieting, but they wouldn't call it depression. The postpartum emotional spectrum comes in many shades. What I have tried to do is describe the range of feelings you may have, while alerting you to the symptoms that are indicative of full-fledged PPD. In the end, labeling our experience PPD or postpartum hormonal hell or a mild case of adjustment blues isn't what matters. What matters is we experience all the unique shadings of what we are feeling, that we never for a moment feel stigmatized if we seek help, and that we have permission to feel whatever we are feeling without feeling guilty or like bad mothers.

General Help

Before we get into individual descriptions of what you may be feeling, check out these ideas for helping yourself feel better emotionally.

Exercise. *If you do nothing else, make time for exercise.* The endorphins that are produced help stimulate your pituitary, which can help naturally regulate the biological components that may be affecting how you are feeling. I know, it may seem impossible to find the time and energy, but it is critical for your well-being. Exercise also helps with anxiety attacks because it helps avoid sudden buildup of lactic acid, a substance that induces these attacks. However, exercising does not mean a two-hour workout. A walk with the baby in a sling on your chest or fifteen minutes of yoga stretches would be perfect.

Talk to other mothers who are willing to discuss openly and honestly what they are feeling.

See Forming Your Support Team; and Resources for help finding moms.

Please don't stay isolated. Isolation makes it worse.

Pay attention to your diet. You still need prenatal vitamins; you may need extra iron (have your hemoglobin checked at your last postnatal visit). Avoid caffeine, alcohol, and sugar as much as you can without making yourself more crazy. Eat small meals like you did when you were pregnant. Frequent amounts of protein can help stabilize mood swings.

Mark your passage. Don't pretend nothing is happening to you. Even if what you are feeling is primarily joyous, and especially when your baby is the most wanted baby on the face of the Earth, you must acknowledge your life's fabric has a new pattern, that things have changed.

Make time every day for true relaxation. That doesn't mean exercising, talking on the phone, painting, or doing anything else that is relaxing. Relaxing means giving your body and mind complete downtime. Become one with the bed. Think of lying on a beach in the warm sun or drifting down a peaceful river on an inner tube.

You need solitude and time to reflect if you are going to create an inner knowing to help you parent and if you are going to remain sane. Make it happen every day. A half hour on the porch with your journal, writing about "I feel . . . ," or a half hour in the tub just letting your mind roll can do wonders for your sanity. Keep your eye on your inner space!

*See Nurturing Yourself
During Pregnancy: Cut to
the Chase for more help.*

Face the importance of making hard choices about your time and energy. If you keep the same pace you did before, you are asking for trouble. Unrealistic and harsh expectations will drive you as crazy as your jittery hormonal balance. Think in terms of a temporary reprieve from perfectionism. It will still be there for you to go back to, don't worry. But for now, let yourself be a slob.

Self-nurturing and support are the very, very best tonics to help you survive and grow during your emergence as a mother. Self-care doesn't have to be a big deal. A little time alone, an aromatic warm bath, a phone conversation with another mother, or hanging around a post-partum exercise class can go a long way toward grounding, giving you a frame of reference. Remember, your needs are as important as the baby's—maybe more important because you have to take care of the baby. You simply cannot care for an infant if you aren't taking care of yourself.

The Emotional Climates

My weather pattern of emotions included: a religious moment on the porch holding Lillian and listening to the mission church bells ringing ("There is a God!"); lots of moments when I was mean enough to eat nails and irrationally angry (I cursed out a lot of innocent people those first few months); a feeling that no one liked me or understood me, that I was ugly, stinky, and strange; elation and enough energy to read three books during breast-feeding the first week; paranoia (I felt that *everyone* blamed Lillian's incessant crying on my being too uptight and intense); waves of aching loneliness ("Why did I move away from all my friends?"); stupendous neediness ("Chris, do you love me? *Why* do you love me? I know you're going to leave me. *Are* you going to leave me?"); and bored isolation.

Name your emotional climate. What are you feeling right now? What were you feeling an hour ago? The day after your baby was born? A week after your child emerged? Make a list in your head or in your journal. Become mindful of your emotional terrain.

Here are a few of the most commonly experienced moods. You may experience something completely different or only a touch of one mood or a combination of many. These descriptions are offered as general guidelines to help you feel less alone.

I'M OPEN WIDE.   Eighty percent of new mothers experience weepiness and sudden mood swings three to ten days after birth. Your hormonal levels *are* plummeting, and that accounts for part of what is making you so tender, but I also believe it is the signal of how you are changing, of how emotionally vulnerable you are going to be for a number of months. You may never feel more exposed, like your heart is always ready to break, like one moment your spirit is big enough to fill the world and the next as fragile and dry as a wishbone withering on your windowsill. Wendy said of her first three weeks, "I kept crying, thinking, 'He's going to grow up so fast.'" Katya couldn't stop telling her husband how wonderful he was, but as soon as she was nursing Max, she would be overcome with intense irritation if her husband came near her.

Consider how your boundaries, physically and psychically, have been laid bare: "Motherhood, particularly late pregnancy, birth, and the first year of a child's life, leave a woman psychologically vulnerable. Her physical resources are continuously being drained with little time for respite and her psychological boundaries are breached in a way that makes her vulnerable to any hint of criticism and rejection and also susceptible to anyone who wishes to 'brainwash' her about how she should behave or what she should be," writes Jane Price in *Motherhood: What It Does to Your Mind.* The psychological defenses with which you protected yourself before are now Swiss cheese, riddled with holes, which makes you incredibly sensitive and incredibly aware.

Treat yourself with kid gloves. Be extraordinarily gentle with yourself. You need a little alone time every day (yes, even if you have other children) so that you can reflect on what you are feeling. Know that the wilder mood swings and weepiness do pass quickly, usually by the end of two weeks. Don't belittle what you are feeling. Try to be open and aware, and, if possible, enjoy it. You may never feel so painfully alive again.

See I'm Open Wide in "Comfort at a Glance" chart for help.

More serious: If you are so depressed or overwhelmed that you can't function, you are experiencing panic or anxiety attacks, or you can't bear the pain, you need to reach out for extra help. See More Help.

I FEEL LIKE I NEED TO BE MOVING, DOING, MOTHERING TWENTY-FOUR HOURS A DAY.   Also known as "I am a mother now and I must nurture everybody at all times." Also known as "I feel so guilty if I'm not doing something twenty-four hours a day." Also known as "I feel guilty no matter what I do." Also known as "Now I'm a mother, I can't be an individual. I am only a mommy."

I am embarrassed to say this one struck me particularly hard. Symptoms include a rabid need to be constantly accomplishing something accompanied by a pounding guilt that you should, must, have to be the only one who cares for the baby. For nine months I had pontificated (boringly) to anyone who would listen about how Chris and I were completely equal partners and how vital it is that a child is raised equally by both parents as well as by other adults. Yet I was sick with guilt when my mother baby-sat Lillian so I could work; when Chris got up and walked her for an hour at 4 A.M.; when I lost my temper with her screaming; when, in any way, I didn't perform heroically and perfectly. The only thing that saved me during this time was Chris's utter astonishment at my behavior and his calm continuance to do what is his right as much as mine: be a parent to his daughter. Chris's attitude, combined with constantly talking to myself with a positive inner voice and nurturing myself in tiny ways, helped me feel less compulsive about my role. I was astonished at how nearly universal and sudden this need always to be doing something was, whether it be handwashing baby clothes (Marilyn), ironing sheets (Jackie), or answering a thank-you note thirty minutes after the gift arrived (me).

Read Nurturing Yourself During Pregnancy; and Isn't Self-Nurturing Impossible with Infants and Toddlers? See Guilt in "Comfort at a Glance" chart.

Solutions? Go on a cruise. Throw back a shot of tequila. Hit yourself repeatedly about the head, neck, and shoulders with a heavy, blunt instrument. Alternative solution: throw away some guilt and take in some self-nurturing.

More serious: If you feel unable to function because you are positive you are doing something wrong or dangerous to your baby, or because you feel completely lacking in self-worth, you need outside support. Refer to More Help.

I'M SO FORGETFUL.   Also called milk brain, baby head, or "I'm so spaced out, I shouldn't be driving." I hated this part so much! My conversations with other people were constantly punctuated with, "I forgot what I was going to say" and "Ummm. What was I saying?" and "What were we talking about?" The inability to complete a thought, to find the right words, or to remember what I had come into the room for, let alone gone to the store for, was maddening. What causes milk brain? Hormonal fluctuations, sleep deprivation, and always feeling preoccupied, as in "Is the baby okay? Am I doing this right?"

Solutions? Get a Hide-a-Key for your car and home. I was incredibly frightened when I thought for a second I had locked Lillian inside a hot car. Be gentle with your loss of memory, your sense of being lost in a fog. Do only one thing at a time, especially if you are having a hard time making decisions. Make little lists aloud: "I am getting some water, then putting on my shoes, then finding the dog's leash, then putting the baby in the pack, then locking the door. Now, I am walking."

See I Am a Body Without a Brain: Practical Advice.

I KEEP IMAGINING ALL OF THESE HORRIBLE THINGS.   You're in the kitchen, your baby in his or her infant seat nearby. You are cutting tomatoes for lunch. You suddenly imagine what it would look like if someone took the knife and cut your baby. You are sickened, appalled, horrified by your imagination, yet you seem powerless to stop your thoughts. Or you are walking with your baby in a stroller across a busy street and you visualize a car running the stoplight and running you over. When your partner doesn't come home on time, you picture graphic accident scenes.

An overactive imagination can be one of the most upsetting reactions to becoming a mother. Your fear is magnified one hundred times over. You can't believe what you find yourself thinking. This pattern is very common. You are not weird. Many of the other mothers around you are entertaining equally ugly and uninvited thoughts. Know that your fear arises partly because you have spent your life being bombarded by horrible, bloody, explicit images of what can happen to a human

Try the thought-stopping techniques in Fear: Controlling Monkey Mind.

being. These fears are being activated by the love that is growing in you for your child, and it is exaggerated by how open you are to everything, both inside and out. Pay attention to your fears, but perform regular reality checks.

More serious: If you are tormented to the point of being sick or experiencing panic attacks, if you are unable to sleep, if when you try to stop yourself you cannot, or if no matter how much you are reassured, you are still frightened something bad is going to happen to your baby, see More Help at the end of this chapter.

MY LIFE WILL NOT CHANGE. You go back to aerobics at two weeks, even though you must hold your uterus in place while you jog. You host a formal dinner party for twenty-five at three weeks postbaby. You return to full-time work at one month, even though you had six weeks' paid leave. You take the baby to Singapore at eight weeks. Then, you collapse. Later, when they let you out of your padded cell, you admit, "My life has changed. I cannot do things in the same way, at the same pace. I see that now." Unfortunately, they don't believe you, and you are locked away for a little more rest.

Your life will never be the same. The best solution for grasping this dizzying, exhilarating, sometimes horrifying truth is to have adjusted your expectations before birth. Barring that, allow yourself to grieve without feeling guilty. The truth is that most of us don't want to stop doing it all. We want our old lives plus our adorable baby. It is so easy to talk about making priorities, but actually saying no to your close friend, giving up exercising every other day when you most want to, and otherwise simplifying your life is hard. It can make you wrathful and woeful. You may be afraid to be housebound, alone with this little being who barely opens his eyes. Or you may be bored, surprised that you are, and perhaps feeling guilty that every minute of motherhood is not fascinating. You may need to pretend your life hasn't changed because you have no one to lean on.

See What's Going to Happen to Me *After the Baby Is Born?; Surrender; and Ambivalence: Grieving the Changes. See also Adjusting Postbaby in the "Comfort at a Glance" chart.*

Try gently examining how much energy you are putting into denying that anything is different (even if you feel you have no choice). If the baby is on the boardroom table in her car seat or out till all hours dancing, it may be time to make a few adjustments. The more energy you put into fighting the change, the harder it will be.

If nothing works, buy a good pair of Rollerblade skates and a backpack for the baby, and keep going. If you need only three hours of sleep, hey, anything is possible.

More serious: If you cannot grasp you have a baby, or feel disconnected from reality, see More Help.

See Tumultuous, Turbulent Feelings for help.

UNBRIDLED JOY, ELATION, HAPPINESS: I HAVE A BABY!   Don't dismiss the surges of intoxicating, transporting ecstasy that can overtake you by saying, "He's smiling now but I know he'll be crying again in a few minutes" or "I still haven't got enough sleep." Luxuriate, wallow, soak up the happy moments! Let the joy in! Break your heart wide open with the sweet, fierce anguish of loving someone this much. It is the essence of being a parent.

More serious: If your mood swings are scaring you, or you find yourself manic with energy one moment, then weeping the next, see More Help.

I AM EXPERIENCING PANIC OR ANXIETY ATTACKS.   A bad panic attack can feel as if you are having cardiac arrest or need to peel your skin off and run screaming through the streets. You may fear you are dying. Your heart races, you may break out in a cold sweat, your limbs can tingle, but, most of all, you are overcome with extreme feelings of panic, dread, and being out of control. A panic attack is truly hell on earth.

If you experience a panic attack more than once, seek outside help. Natural (not synthetic) progesterone injections can be very helpful. You also should have your thyroid checked, which involves a simple blood test.

THERE ARE MOMENTS WHEN I HATE MY BABY.   The baby has been screaming for hours or what seems like hours. You're singing yet another senseless lullaby. Her face is purple. Nothing you do makes any difference. Suddenly, you are filled with a heat wave of fury, and you can see yourself hurling the baby across the room.

The first time this happened to me, I was trying (and failing) to soothe Lillian at 3 A.M. As I was walking and bouncing her, I found myself bouncing her just a little bit hard. I was immediately overcome with shame and fear. I was sure this one bounce meant I had a predilection for child abuse. I knew I was doomed to be a horrible, cold, withdrawn mother from now on to avoid hurting my own child. As I sat alone in my house in the middle of the night and sobbed, I had never felt more wormlike or despicable in my life.

I dared to mention this intense anger to Alice, a midwife and mother of two. It was so utterly wonderful to hear her say, "Yes, that is horrible. And scary. I hated it when I have felt that way." I wasn't alone! I wasn't insane! I wouldn't have to pay for fifteen years of analysis for my daughter (well, at least not yet).

It is common to feel almost overwhelming anger at your tiny infant. Sleep deprivation combined with feeling out of control and helpless ("Why can't I get her to stop crying?"), isolation, and perhaps your own unconscious memories of being a dependent, frustrated infant make your rage so desperate. Put the baby down in the bassinet, even if he or she is wailing, step outside in your bare feet, and feel the Earth under your toes. Forgive yourself. Hug your dog or cat if you have one. *Get someone else to take care of the baby for even fifteen minutes, but a few hours is best.* Call your local hospital and see if it has a warm line or a women's resource center where someone trained in these situations can reassure you what you are feeling is normal. Get a massage to release tension. Scream in the shower.

See I Want My Mommy for some self-mothering suggestions; and But Isn't Self-Nurturing Impossible with Infants and Toddlers? for self-loving suggestions.

It is imperative that you don't let your anger spiral you into a cycle of self-hatred. This will batter your self-esteem into a pulp and steal your confidence as a mother. Forgive yourself. Talk to other mothers. Nurture yourself.

More serious: If you often feel close to hurting, compelled to hurt, or obsessed with the thought that you will hurt yourself or your baby, get help immediately. See the introduction of this section for crisis suggestions and Resources for information numbers to call. If you are at all worried you have crossed the line, get help *now*.

I AM FILLED WITH REGRET AND LOSS.   Summer twilight fills your living room as you pace with your newborn. She fusses and then screams and then sucks on the pacifier and then fusses and adds a few piercing screams for good measure. You stand at your window and watch the world going by: a couple jogging, a young woman walking her dog, neighbors drinking wine on their deck. You feel like a kid forced to go to bed while your friends still play outside. And it is all the baby's fault.

As unmotherly and shocking as feelings of remorse and grief are, they are as natural and inevitable as the labor that brought this being into your arms. Feelings of loss are one of strongest, most common, and less sanctioned feelings new moms experience. It doesn't matter how much you wanted your baby or how long you waited or how much you went through to get pregnant. No one can prepare herself for the impact, the life-wrenching change, of a baby, especially a first child (but often a second has an equally meteoric effect). The regrets will be mixed with love and will fade with time, although they tend to rear their heads now and then, especially if you run into an old boyfriend while wearing baggy sweats covered with spit-up.

Our inability as a culture to talk honestly about the changes a baby brings—our insistence on focusing on only the positive—can leave us feeling despicable if we dare mention the moments we don't like having a baby. But when we don't allow ourselves to grieve and talk about the adjustments honestly, to "embrace the change instead of denying it," as critical care pediatric nurse Marilyn Downy said, we may experience these losses as depression. Or as psychologist Brad Sachs points out, if we are troubled by aspects of motherhood, we are tempted to overfunction and keep moving, to shove our feelings away to avoid discomfort. We slip with a sigh into that broken-down, uncomfortable, but oh-so-familiar pair of running shoes, the ones that allow us to be indispensable, to take care of others and not stop to figure out what we are feeling.

We must make it okay to talk about the shadow side of becoming a mother. The only way to do that is to open your mouth and start naming how you feel to another mother. Consider writing in your

See Ambivalence: Grieving
the Changes for grieving
guidelines; and What's
Going to Happen to Me
After the Baby Is Born?
for help remembering who
you are.

journal about why it isn't okay to have regrets and mourn having a baby. Who said it isn't okay? What scares you about feeling this way? Do you believe if you admit you are sad it means you don't love your baby? Are you afraid that if you admit motherhood isn't perfect, it means your mother didn't love you? Contemplate these questions. Another good journal exercise is to make a list of all the things you miss about your old life before this baby. Be specific and detailed. Let go on paper.

The desire to grieve and to name your losses may seem selfish and irrelevant to you right now. Fine. Be aware, however, if you experience the onset of a low-grade, creeping depression, perhaps at eight or nine months postbaby, you may need to grieve then.

More serious: If you are unable to stop crying or control your crying or you are so depressed or despondent you can't care for your baby or yourself, you are beyond what you should try to handle alone. See More Help.

I'M NOT BONDING WITH MY BABY. The pressure to love your baby the moment it arrives is very, very strong. Any mother who takes a few days, weeks, let alone months to fall in love can feel sorrowful, ashamed, worthless: basically pond scum. I wish I could hold your hand and tell you, "You will love your baby. You are going through a cataclysmic adaptation. Be patient, talk to someone who understands, and relax." You will look back on this time and smile. Or at least breathe a sigh of relief. You are forming a new relationship. Babies come out, and each of us must learn how to be a mother, how to be in relationship with this creature of our blood. This will be the most intimate relationship of your life. If it takes a while to warm up to that or figure out how to proceed, that's perfectly normal.

See What's Going to
Happen to Me After the
Baby Is Born?: The Myth
of the Perfect Mother.

Some women love it when their baby is an infant; others do much better with other stages. "Overall, mothers who had difficulty handling the stresses of infancy were no more likely to have negative relationships with their children in the long run than those who found infancy thoroughly rewarding. From a mother's point of view, feeling complete love toward one's infant is not crucial to loving one's child deeply later on," note Louis Genevie and Eva Margolies in *The Mother-hood Report*. It is okay that having a baby isn't the most incredible thing that has ever happened to you so far. If you find you are truly hating this stage, if at all possible seek a substitute caregiver. If your mate is more nurturing than you right now, let him or her do the cooing and tickling. Recognize your strengths and your weaknesses, but refuse to be cowed by a saccharine, limited view of motherhood.

More serious: If you can't touch your baby without feeling overcome with revulsion or guilt, see More Help.

I FEEL LET DOWN AND FORGOTTEN.   When you anticipate something for most of a year, and then it happens, you are bound to feel a wee wave of disappointment. This feeling of being disregarded is exacerbated by the tremendous amount of attention you receive just prior to and following the birth. People who haven't contacted you in years emerge, pestering, "Have you had it yet?" But after a few weeks, the UPS truck doesn't stop at your door anymore, the phone doesn't ring because people don't want to bother you, and isolation can set in like ice cloaking a lake in winter.

Planning ahead is the best insurance. *But it is never too late to reach out for contact.* If you can, ask one close friend to call you once a week and ask about you only. Tell her or him if you want to talk about the baby, you'll bring it up. If you can afford it, order something from a catalog so a package comes for you. (Join a book club with a free starter offer.) Ask another friend to surprise you over the next few weeks with a couple of silly cards or postcards. Dredge up anyone you can think of that you haven't sent birth announcements to, then hope they call or send gifts. Find a new mothers' group. You don't have to go, but knowing there is contact when you have the energy can be reassuring.

See Forming Your Support Team; and Adjusting Postbaby in the "Comfort at a Glance" chart for more suggestions.

More serious: If you feel so isolated you find it too difficult to have even the most basic conversation with someone you are close to, or if you wonder if the people around can tell you are going crazy, you need to talk to someone. It may be almost impossible for you to reach out. Choose carefully whom you reach out to. If possible, make it one of the phone numbers in the Resource section, unless there is someone close to you who will understand. The first contact is the hardest, but if you can make that initial call, or have someone make it for you, you will not regret it. Read More Help first.

I FEEL LIKE I FAILED AT THE BIRTH.   If you had a C-section, bellowed for an epidural, offered to sell your baby for drugs, or just wanted to be left alone to sleep after the delivery (instead of cooing over your new-born), you may be experiencing a feeling of having failed to be a real woman and experience the life-changing, spiritually ecstatic reverence of birth.

See the next section, "I Feel Fat and Dowdy," and Postbirth Nourishment: Surviving and Thriving: Recovering Emotionally from an Unplanned Cesarean Birth for suggestions that can be translated to this situation.

A backlash of the movement to put birth back into women's hands has been the propagation of the idea that any woman who doesn't give birth quietly, gracefully, and without drugs and who doesn't instantly adore her baby has failed. Too many people have forgotten that each woman is unique and that birth is a mystery. Your genes, your body type, the father's body type, your past experience with birth, where you give birth—all of these affect your labor, and many are completely beyond your control. Don't forget the baby; it is very likely that tiny human has a lot to do with when your labor starts and how it unfolds. You can be the best-prepared woman, the least fearful, the most fit in the world and still suffer extraordinary pain and unforeseen complications. Labor and delivery are the final preparation for parenting: you must surrender to the unpredictable, the mystery.

More serious: If after several weeks, when you are with your child, all you can think about is how you failed, or if you find yourself dieting strictly, purging after a meal, or in any way punishing yourself, see More Help.

I FEEL FAT AND DOWDY.   It is so heart-wrenchingly sad that after nourishing a life inside ourselves and bringing that life into the world, after caressing that silky peewee face and sucking on those luscious Lilliputian toes, we still find ourselves disappointed with our bodies. Moaning about our soft, squishy bellies. Avoiding the mirror. Surreptitiously slipping into our khakis or suit skirts, hoping they will button, and gnashing our teeth when they don't. Wasting precious moments obsessing over our weight. What will it take to revere our womanly form, to pay homage to the body that has created life?

Create a thank-your-body ritual or, as Anne Lamott says, "an awards ceremony" for your body. Find a moonlit patch of Earth, lie down naked, and let the moonlight caress your limbs as you whisper your thanks. Or go skinny-dipping (the tub will suffice in winter months) and imagine the water is lapping a thank-you all over you. Or anoint yourself with oil and massage your belly, visualizing how it helped you grow your child. Anoint your arms and thank them for letting you hold your baby. Bless each part of your body for how it helped you make your baby or how it will help you love your child. Or sit in a circle of candles and recite to your higher power all the reasons your body is holy. Or visit a shrine in nature or a church and thank God/Goddess for your functioning body.

The more pragmatic might try these ideas:

Store and return borrowed maternity clothes as soon as possible.

Put in your closet only the clothes that you can wear now. The rest can go in another closet, paper bags, or a box under the bed. As you slim down, introduce "new" clothes.

Shop for shoes. Unless even your feet feel fat.

Shop for or decorate one part of your body you like. A pedicure and new sandals if you love your feet, a rub-on tattoo for a shoulder (just because you are a mother doesn't mean you have to be boring), an intensive hair conditioner, a fabulous new hat.

Collect images of robust mothers with their children. Visit a museum gift shop or woman's bookstore. Tack the images up everywhere.

If you need new clothes, shop through catalogs. It's much less depressing than seeing yourself in those fluorescent purgatory changing rooms—and you don't have to hire a baby-sitter.

See Comforting Clothing and Other Sensual Strategies.

Every time you despair, remember your extra flesh has served an invaluable purpose. Feel the phenomenal sensuous delight you take in your baby's body, and then transfer a little of that to your own body. How many times do you say to your baby, "I just want to eat you up?" Let that love of the physical rub off on you. Look at your thighs and then look at your baby's thighs. You don't find her extra flesh ugly, you find it rosy and scrumptious. You are still as perfect and beautiful as your baby. Really. Attempt to believe this for a split second.

More serious: If you are breast-feeding and trying to diet strictly, if you spend an inordinate amount of time bemoaning how horrible you look, if you check the scale after every meal, or if you are suffering from an eating disorder, see More Help.

I CAN'T LEAVE MY CHILD. Separation anxiety is common and heart wrenching. It is often felt the most searingly by working moms upon returning to work. Leaving your baby with a baby-sitter for the first time can also be excruciating. The whole time you are away, you feel you are missing an appendage. You may find yourself imagining you hear your baby crying in the distance. If you spend the night away from your baby, you may wake up looking for him or her in the bed covers or bathroom.

You are feeling this way because your very core is being drenched with love. You are experiencing the pay-off of parenthood, the good stuff, what everyone tries to describe when they talk about how stupendous it is to have kids. You are also experiencing yourself as a separate individual. The early weeks of motherhood are a time of intense merging. Your baby does not know yet where he ends and you begin. To a lesser degree, you experience the same blurring of boundaries. This merging is healthy for both of you. It is what helps you fall in love with your baby. But at some point, it is healthy for you to step back and reassert your boundaries. This too is an important part of being a mother. However, it can be painful.

Don't force yourself. It may be months before you can feel comfortable being away from your child. Have someone watch your baby while you nurture yourself in another part of your home. When you first leave your child, be sure it is with someone you trust completely, like your partner, your mother, sister, or best friend. Make your first outing short; have a very simple and specific place to go. Work your way up to several hours away from home. When you feel ready to leave your baby with someone new, first hire this person to baby-sit while you stay home (perhaps to have friends over for a potluck or to take a nap). Use only a baby-sitter whom a friend has used or who comes from a bonded service.

If you are unable to leave your child at all, you may need some professional help to deal with your own fears of abandonment. Your inability to separate may affect your child, making it harder for him or her to individuate. Talk to someone.

If you have a partner, be aware that your mate might not be able to understand your inability to leave and might feel neglected and jealous. These are legitimate feelings too. If you are very focused on your child, it can be hard on your relationship. Don't be harsh on yourself if you love being with your infant, and be clear that you aren't responsible for your mate's feelings. But don't use your new love affair as an excuse to neglect yourself or your relationship either.

More serious: If you experience anxiety or panic attacks beyond the first time or two you leave your child with someone besides your partner or a relative, see More Help.

I'm SLEEP DEPRIVED.   Do not underestimate the power of sleep deprivation to make you completely deranged. Researchers in the field of PPD feel the role sleep deprivation plays in causing or worsening depression has been minimized. It will cause you to feel prickly with irritation, unable to bear the slightest extra strain. (When I was exhausted and walked into the kitchen to find the counters black with ants parading everywhere, I lost it.) You may have a hard time thinking through and performing the simplest tasks. Your baby's crying can set your nerves on edge almost instantly, making you feel repulsive for not being more patient. You could feel completely undone by the smallest change in your routine.

You must get some uninterrupted sleep. Do not see this as an unachievable luxury. It is your human right, and it is an organic part of your mental health. Be aware you might feel great for the first few weeks or even months and then crash (going back to work can send women over the edge). Your partner returning to work or a helper returning

See But Isn't Self-Nurturing Impossible with Infants and Toddlers?: Practical Ideas for Overcoming Guilt. For help with anxiety, see Anxiety in the "Comfort at a Glance" chart.

See Postbirth Nourishment: Surviving and Thriving: Sleep for suggestions.

home leaves you open to a new level of fatigue. You must make sleep your number one priority.

More serious: Because so many of the symptoms identified with PPD can also be caused by sleep deprivation, the only way to know the difference is to get sleep. It is possible if you are willing to reach out and perhaps demand help.

If you are suffering from insomnia, you may need extra help. See More Help.

See Appendix: Herbs, Oils, and Other Natural Comforters for recipes for better sleep.

More Help: Postpartum Depression

If you are feeling too much pain, confusion, or depression to cope, if you are struggling with any of the symptoms listed above under "More serious," or if you simply feel overwhelmed and unsure of what to do, *there is help available*—wonderful, loving, nonshaming, effective help.

Know that:

Things will get better. PPD is completely treatable. You are not weird, alone, or a horrible mother. Postpartum depression is very complex and is far from being completely understood. It is a condition best called "biopsychosocial": it has as much to do with your rapidly slowing down endocrine system (bio) as it does your mental state (psycho) and the high expectations and isolation imposed on new mothers (social). The fall in estrogen you experience after delivery can affect the function of your pituitary gland; the pituitary is the gland that secretes the myriad of hormones controlling other glands, like your thyroid and adrenals—glands that produce substances affecting your emotions. This combined with the stress and often-unexpected adjustment to your new baby, as well as the lack of support for mothers in our society, probably triggers PPD. Because so little research has been done on the condition, no one knows its exact causes.

The sooner you get help, the sooner you will recover. Delaying seeking help can allow your depression to deepen and make your recovery longer and more complicated.

The worst myth about PPD is that it hits only women who are neurotic, who don't want their babies, who have careers, or women who are predisposed to depression and mental health problems. This is a lie. Women from all walks of life, all ages, and all sorts of life situations get PPD. No one knows why one woman gets it and another doesn't. The only generally agreed upon factors are the lack of support mothers experience in our culture, the mandate that women must put their needs behind everyone else's, and the subsequent lack of nurturing postpartum (including sleep deprivation).

To get help:

You must reach out. The stigma surrounding mental health difficulties must not stop you from feeling better. The sooner you talk to someone who understands PPD, the sooner you are going to get relief. Don't try to cope alone. There is no need to. Please, please reach out for help.

It is still difficult to find proper, compassionate, up-to-date treatment for PPD. Many doctors don't recognize the seriousness of PPD. Other doctors do but fail to take a multifaceted approach to caring for you. PPD is different from any other disorder. You must receive treatment that takes into account what is happening to you physically, psychologically, and socially. If only one aspect is treated, the treatment may not work. For instance, if you see a psychotherapist who wants to talk only about your childhood and how that relates to being a mother, you may end up feeling worse. What you need now more than anything is reassurance, support for what you are experiencing, and help getting your hormones back on track.

To find help, call one of the numbers listed below in Resources. Call with any questions or concerns about how you are feeling. If you feel too depressed to call, have someone else call for you. The people at these organizations are wonderful; they will do everything they can to help you find the proper care in your area, which could include short-term psychotherapy with someone who is familiar with PPD, hormonal therapy (try to insist on naturally produced progesterone), nutritional advice, help creating a support system while you recover, and especially the name of a PPD support group nearest you or the telephone number of a someone who has recovered. Just talking about what you are going through with someone who has been there can be tremendously helpful.

You can also find help by calling your local birth or parents' resource center, a women's resource center (look for these at local colleges, universities, or hospitals), or a new mothers' support group for recommendations. Or ask your health care provider or your pediatrician to recommend a therapist. Church clergy can be another good source. If someone does make a recommendation, be sure to ask if he or she has gotten feedback from anyone previously referred.

Have your thyroid checked. Too many women have experienced agonizing depression and faulty treatment when a simple blood test and subsequent medication would have quickly corrected the situation. Insist even if your doctor doesn't want to.

You are most vulnerable to the onset of PPD in the first two weeks following the birth of your baby, in the first two weeks before you resume your period, and in the two weeks following weaning your child.

If medication is prescribed, it doesn't mean you are insane or "really sick." It simply means you have a pattern of symptoms that suggests you will respond well to medication. The choice is always yours. Be informed. Take an active, consumer approach. Learn about the drug you are taking; read *The Physician's Desk Reference* for the drug you are prescribed. Be aware you must be carefully monitored. If someone suggests giving you a drug and seeing you again in a month, it isn't okay. A month is a very long time in your life right now. Insist on being seen in a week. Also be aware that taking medication doesn't mean you must stop breast-feeding. Insist on finding out what drugs you could take that would allow you to continue, if you wish to.

The most important thing to remember is if you feel like you need help, get it. Please, please don't be imprisoned by the ridiculous idea that you should somehow be able to cope all on your own, that you are a failure as a woman if you reach out.

Resources:

The following centers are volunteer staffed, compassionate, and experienced. None are twenty-four hours. Even if you aren't sure you have PPD, don't hesitate to call.

Depression After Delivery, P.O. Box 1282, Morrisville, PA 19067. Phone, in the U.S., 800-944-4773. If you leave your address, you will be promptly mailed a packet of information. DAD sponsors chapters and local support people all over the country. http://www.depressionafterdelivery.com

Postpartum Support International, 927 North Kellogg Avenue, Santa Barbara, CA 93111. Phone 805-967-7636. PSI is Jane Honkiman's labor of love. Her role is to "make the mother feel number one and reaffirm her importance," and she does a wonderful job of doing just that. http://www.postpartum.net

Postpartum Mood Disorders Clinic, 6635 Crawford Street, San Diego, CA 92129. The clinic provides a brochure on PPD and a networking list to provide local referrals for women around the country.

In Canada:

Aid for New Mothers, P.O. Box 84, Station M, Ontario, Toronto M6S 4T2, Canada. Phone 416-535-2368. Resources include a list of services throughout Canada, packet on PPD, and local telephone support, referrals, support group, and one-on-one counseling.

Books:

Big Purple Mommy: Nurturing Our Creative Work, Our Children, and Ourselves, by Coleen Hubbard (The Berkeley Publishing Group, 2001)

Child of Mine: Original Essays on Becoming a Mother, by Christina Baker Kline (Dell Publishing, 1997)

Little Moments of Peace: Daily Reflections for Mothers, by Andrea Gosline (Penguin Putnam Tarcher, 2002). I wish I had this book when I was a young mother.

Meditations for New Mothers, by Beth Wilson Saavedra (Workman, 1992). Just about every emotional state is covered in Saavedra's reassuring book.

Mother Nurture, by Rick Hanson, Jan Hanson, and Ricki Pollycove (Penguin, 2002). Help with parenting, lowering stress, increasing energy, lifting your mood, building teamwork with your mate, and staying intimate friends with each other.

Mothering the New Mother, by Sally Placksin (Newmarket Press, 2000). Good overview section on PPD, excellent list of resources, including local support groups and clinics.

Mothers Who Think: Tales of Real-Life Parenthood, edited by Camille Peri, Kate Moses, Daphne Marneffe, Anne Lamott (Washington Square Press, 2000). Funny! Honest! Smart!

Special Momease™ Designed as a much-needed soother for the newly born mother, this kit is a wonderful way for any woman to take a few moments for herself. Includes music, journal, aromatherapies and other amenities for babying the other baby. Find out where to buy at http://www.fortyweeks.com

The Blue Jay's Dance: A Birth Year, by Louise Erdrich (Harper, 1995). Poetic.

The Happiest Baby on the Block: The New Way to Calm Crying and Help Your Baby Sleep Longer, by Harvey Karp, MD (Bantam, 2003). A new method to calm and soothe babies.

The Mother's Well-Being Book, by Lisa Goren Braner (Conari Press, 2003). A mother's comfort book—highly recommended!

The Woman's Book of Yoga and Health: A Lifelong Guide to Wellness, by Linda Sparrowe, Patricia Walden, and Judith Hanson Lasater (Shambhala, 2002). Yoga for post-birth help and hormonal balancing.

This Isn't What I Expected, by Karen R. Kleiman, M.S.W., and Valerie D. Raskin, M.D. (Bantam, 1994). The very best book on the subject of postpartum depression. If you are experiencing any of the "More Serious" symptoms or are feeling at all out of it, get this book! Contains a rundown of the different medications and side effects.

Websites:

She Knows
http://SheKnows.com

Nurture Mom
http://www.NurtureMom.com

LiteraryMama.com
http://www.literarymama.com

Receiving the Nurturing You Need from Your Partner Postpartum (and Giving a Little Too)

When to Do It:

- Immediately following the baby's birth.

- If when you look at your partner, you can't remember his or her name.

- When all your conversations are about sleep or lack of it, time and amount of last poop, or spit-up velocity, except when you discuss scintillating topics like travel arrangements for visiting in-laws or quibble over who paid the bills late.

What Is It?

The baby lies there crying and all you want to do is lie down and wail too. You want someone to feed you, tuck you into bed, make the world whole and safe. The logical person for mothers in partnerships is your mate. Single moms may feel this need for nurturing even more strongly, which is why your support system must include someone you can be vulnerable and needy with: a best friend, brother, sister, or your mother. You need a tremendous amount of love, attention, and compassion right now.

Having a baby reminds you of what it was like to be a baby. It awakens your own desire to be dependent and taken care of and can also bring

You'll Need:

Snatches of time daily with your mate.

Occasional two hours or more of time sans infant.

A tiny bit of mad money.

childhood issues to the forefront. Yet if you have a partner who is helping to raise the baby, your mate will have needs and desires of his or her own. Your relationship has needs too, if it is to stay alive and healthy. But nurturing each other and your relationship is difficult under the best of circumstances. It is almost impossible with a new baby. That *almost* offers the slimmest shimmer of hope that you will find the time and energy to stay in contact and get the support you so need right now.

What to Do:

Why Your Mate Needs Nurturing and Understanding from You

For women in heterosexual partnerships, it helps to understand how your mate may be feeling. Having a baby may make him feel needy and vulnerable too, but these are uncomfortable feelings for a man to have, let alone acknowledge. He receives little attention or support; few people ask how he is feeling, how the baby is affecting his life. He may want to be babied and cared for by you. This often manifests itself as a desire for sex, which probably interests you about as much as going through labor again. You may find yourself resenting his need for attention and reassurance because you are giving twenty-four hours a day to your baby. Your mate may also feel like competing with your newborn for your nurturance and love. Add a dash of sleep deprivation, work responsibilities crowding in, and, of course, the baby, who is getting everybody's time, attention, and nurturing. Doesn't sound like there will be a lot of energy left for champagne and edible underwear.

If Your Partner is a Woman

Women in same-sex partnerships will find themselves dealing with many of the same relationship issues, although it is less common for the nonbiological mother to feel competitive toward the baby. Yet if the biological mother chooses to breast-feed, it can leave the other partner feeling especially left out, as in "My body could do that too."

It helps if the mom who isn't breast-feeding can be the primary person to do certain things, like bathing or rocking in the middle of the night (every partner should have his or her fair share of sleep deprivation).

Nurturing Ideas for Needy Partners

Postbaby relationship stress is normal! It doesn't mean you are headed for trouble. Everyone experiences tension, moments of meltdown, (often along with greater intimacy and commitment), less sex or no sex, no patience with each other, and, above all, the need to be taken care of. Be assured you are normal if you suddenly hate the person you've had this baby with, if you come unraveled over your mate eating the last of the double chocolate chunk banana ice cream. However, doing everything you can (which won't be much since your energy levels are so low) to keep in contact will minimize the pain and perhaps maximize the joy.

Keep in mind you both need love, attention, validation, approval, help, and relief during these first few months. Post these words on your bulletin board or refrigerator.

Forget about taking care of anyone else outside the relationship. Be relentless and merciless in cutting your life to the minimum. Don't waste precious energy entertaining people who want to see the baby or keeping up social engagements. You must protect each other. Yes, you will lose friends. It is going to happen anyway. It is a reflection of how your life is changing. You must use your time very, very carefully now, and people and hobbies will have to fall by the wayside.

In the first few weeks, especially weeks three through six, each of you can ask yourself, "How do I need to be nurtured?" Do this while you are feeding the baby or taking a shower. Share what you discover. Support each other to act on your ideas or to do for each other what is needed. For example, if you discover you need more sleep to feel nurtured (you will!), your mate can watch the baby on Saturday while you nap or help you hire a preteen to watch the baby while you nap together. If your partner discovers he or she needs more sex to feel nurtured and that isn't good for you right now, you can partially meet this need by giving a five-minute back massage. You won't be able to nurture yourself or each other every time (not by a long shot), but by identifying and communicating your ideas, you stay in much closer touch with each other.

Having a child can stir up childhood traumas and fears. If either you or your partner is adopted, is a survivor of incest, grew up in an alcoholic or violent family, or experienced early trauma, be aware that the first year is prime time for these old issues to spring up. The good news is each of you has an opportunity to heal, again or for the first time, and the healing often occurs quickly. The difficult news is you will have fewer reserves of energy and patience, fewer defenses, to protect you. *Please* be willing to seek outside help.

Don't discount sleep deprivation. If you find yourself bursting into tears when you spill your coffee, you aren't going crazy. Don't blame yourself and don't hold it against your partner. Just keep repeating, "We will get through this. It doesn't last forever."

Gatekeeping

"Don't leave her alone on the changing table" and "He doesn't like to be held that way, he likes to be held this way," are examples of gatekeeping, a term used to describe the ways one parent "knows best" and blocks, frustrates, or invalidates the other parent from participating in raising the child. Gatekeeping can be particularly strong if your infant was premature or had health problems. Child development guru T. Berry Brazelton writes in his book *Touchpoints,*

> All adults who care about a baby will naturally be in competition for that baby. Competitive feelings are a normal component of caring for a dependent individual. Each adult wishes that he or she could do each job a bit more skillfully for the infant or small child than the other.

Some gatekeeping is inevitable, healthy, and a sign that each parent cares about the baby.

What you want to avoid, from the very beginning, is excessive gate-keeping. Because women are supposed to be natural experts on children, because mothers are supposed to be selfless and do it all, we can fall into the trap of excessive gatekeeping. By doing so we strengthen these imprisoning assumptions and rob our partners of the confidence they need to be good parents. We make ourselves indispensable, which means we never get time off. In addition, we can erode the relationship between partner and child, a relationship that has an equally valid right to exist and needs to be equally vital.

Be warned: gatekeeping is very, very tempting. T. Berry Brazelton goes on to write about a full-time dad who brought his daughter to all her checkups. Brazelton marveled at the mother's ability to sit back and let Dad take over. "However, I also found myself worrying about her own attachment to the baby. Later, I realized this reaction came from my stereotyped expectation of what mothers should do," he confessed. Most of us have that same stereotype working inside of us. Gate-keeping makes us feel useful, intelligent, sure of ourselves in our new, fragile role. It also has a lot to do with doing with what we think we should be doing, what others expect of us as moms.

"While the modern mother is constantly told by her forebears how fortunate she is to raise children in an era in which men help out so willingly, she still tends to feel threatened by this help rather than appreciative of it. She smiles weakly when her child calls for Daddy rather than Mommy at night, . . . " notes Brad Sachs in his book, *Things Just Haven't Been the Same.* The majority of us still get our womanhood confirmed on the deepest level by our ability to nurture and care for our offspring. We feel instinctively that we will be devalued and rejected if we share our nurturing role with our mates. This belief is often hidden, hard to lay our hands on, because we may also believe in equal partnerships. But if we fail to be conscious of how we react to our partners helping, if we don't query ourselves about whether we honestly want our babies to grow into people who want their daddies as much as their mommies, we will send contradictory and confusing messages to our partners about sharing responsibility. So as you step back and bite your tongue, check with your heart to see what it is saying about sharing your baby. It may take time to hear the reply. You may feel guilty and confused; you may feel an ache in your arms. Simply be conscious. Don't stop yourself from searching your soul by saying, "It's a moot point! He wouldn't do his share anyway!" That is a separate issue, one that cannot be settled until you are clear about how much you want to share your baby.

Don't assume you are completely exonerated from this tug-of-war if you are in a lesbian partnership. Hope that the baby will want you just a *little* bit more than her and the belief that you know best how to mother can exist in the most radical feminist's heart. In addition, these beliefs can make you feel ashamed. "I'm a lesbian, I'm not supposed to feel this way." Forget politics and share your heart with your mate.

Suggestions for minimizing gatekeeping:

- Ask your mate to read the same child-rearing books you read. If he or she is "too busy," highlight the most important passages. This gives you both the same knowledge base and eliminates the need for you to be the expert.

- Try very hard to attend the first three pediatrician visits together. Have your partner attend a visit alone.

*See Postbirth
Nourishment: Surviving
the Emotions: I Can't
Leave My Child.*

*See Sharing Your
Doubts below.*

- Leave your partner alone with the baby *from the very beginning*. Don't hover, don't give advice. If you have to leave the house or have a glass of wine to do so, fine.

- Share your fears about doing something wrong, about hurting your child, about not being a good parent. Be as specific and honest as you can about your own inadequacies. Gatekeeping gets worse the more you pretend to be the perfect parent.

Other adults will also gatekeep. The hottest topic is breast-feeding, with advice coming from grandparents or aunts or sisters who did not. "How do you know you have enough milk?" or "Maybe she would sleep better if you gave her formula" or "It wouldn't hurt to just try a little formula" are favorite quotes. This kind of gatekeeping can be a grinding source of frustration and can quickly rob both of you of any modicum of parenting self-confidence. The best approach is to respond with, "I know you care about the baby. I'll take your suggestion into consideration." Then, when you are by yourself or alone with your mate, consider the suggestion calmly, trying to tune in to what your inner wisdom says is right. Ninety-five percent of the advice you will throw out. The rest you can incorporate, but from a place of trusting and judging yourself, not grabbing at straws or pleasing others. And if this tactic fails (as it may), let loose an earsplitting howl, rip hair from your head, fall to your knees slobbering, and beg the other person to shut up. Then, stand up, calmly wipe your mouth, and say something like, "Those pesky hormones. They sure can make a gal crazy." (When trapped, resort to using biology to wriggle free.)

Sharing Your Doubts

Regularly, maybe once a week, take five minutes to voice to each other all the ways you think you've screwed up as a parent recently. Indulge each other's emotions. Tune in to your critical voice, which has such fun pointing out all your terrible flaws. Take turns. For example:

You: The baby is only crying because I am so uptight.

Your partner: I am already not paying enough attention to her. I am going to be just as preoccupied as my father was.

You: She's angry at me because I leave her and go to work. I'm not bonded to her enough.

Your partner: I'm never here either. I'm already the absent father, and she's only four weeks old!

End with a hug or a "Thanks for showing me your demons."

Don't react to your partner's statements, even with positive feedback. If you do, it tends to minimize your mate's particular brand of self-flagellation, and he or she won't feel heard. Share your doubts without comment. This deflates the devils, allowing you to be vulnerable with each other as parents. If you want to reassure your mate about a particular statement, do so the next day. However, don't hesitate to hug, grin, and otherwise comfort each other.

Another useful way to stay in contact is to name the sacrifices you aren't enjoying making, to name the ways you are finding being a parent not so great. Use the same system, taking turns trading your most wicked and petty complaints.

For example:

You: All I want to do is take a shower, alone, without her crying halfway through.

Your partner: I want eight hours' sleep. I demand eight hours' sleep!

You: I hate not being able to drop everything and go to a movie.

Your partner: I despise feeling trapped.

End by exchanging a positive statement like "I love you and I know you love our child, even if you hate being a parent sometimes."

Of course, you can also communicate what you cherish about being a parent. Take turns before bed or on your way out for a date to impart "happiness hiccups," those usually sudden moments with your child when time stands still, your heart exults with joy, and you know why you are a parent. Too often these slip past without comment, and when we are with our partners we focus on the problems—on how to get her to sleep or him to eat. Stopping to remember the good moments helps sear them into our memories and lighten the load.

Nurture the Child in Each Other

Because having a child makes us feel like a child, sometimes the most effective way to nurture each other is to acknowledge the childlike parts in each other. Encourage and allow each other dependent time. Baby each other. That might mean serving him coffee in bed or rubbing her back as she goes to sleep or making him mashed potatoes or lying on the bed together, making baby noises and kicking your legs and arms in air (a real-life example that purportedly works miracles). Don't judge each other for acting babyish or needing one another. Try:

- Drawing a bath for your partner.

- Tucking your mate into bed.

- Rocking your partner in your lap.

- Putting chocolates on her pillow.

- Doing a household responsibility you know he hates, like buying the groceries, paying the rent, or cleaning the litter box.

- Folding the laundry the way her mother did.

- Together, buying or cooking favorite childhood foods, like tuna casserole, Neapolitan ice cream, Jell-O with miniature marshmallows.

- Asking each other, "When are the grown-ups coming home?"

Give Each Other Time Alone

Sometime after the birth, a power struggle begins to arise between you and your partner—not over the baby but over who gets time alone, time to enjoy themselves, time to veg out. Mutual feelings of being deprived of freedom and private time can have you at each other's throats.

Try designating one or two nights a week as your nights on duty and one or two nights as your partner's and one night as couple night. The weekends are family time. In addition, you can give each other chunks of time on the weekends, alternating Saturday afternoons, for example. This system won't work until your infant has settled into a schedule, especially if you are breast-feeding. However, even early on, you can be off-duty between feedings. When you are off-duty, you don't have to leave the house. You might choose to play with the child(ren), hang out with your mate, or do chores, but the choice is yours. You get to do only what you want. By declaring ahead of time who is on and who is off, when you want to read the paper on the porch, you don't have to feel guilty whey baby starts to wail. You can truly relax. Note: You must decide at what time child duty starts and stops. Does it start after dinner and dishes? Does it go all night long, meaning that person gets up with the baby? Spell it out realistically and clearly.

This system implies a neat, clean, orderly world. This is never the case. The system won't always work. Your partner will have to travel for business, leaving you for a week with the baby every day and night. If you don't work outside the home you might need more than two nights off a week; you will need a week off at some point! Just keep in mind the baby is both parents' responsibility. The more you can believe that, the better. Second, forget tit for tat. Sometimes one person is going to need more time off—for sanity or work. Give him or her that time without expecting anything in return. Your lover will feel honestly nurtured, and you can rest assured, in the eighteen-some years your child will be with you, you will have plenty of opportunity to ask for your own time. Take the long view. Note: This doesn't mean you shouldn't stand up for yourself if you feel the division of labor is unfair.

The Witching Hour

Almost every couple has trouble with the transition between work and home. If you stay home, you often have a desperate need for relief by the time your mate comes in the door. But that parent has also had a hard day out in the world and may crave a little silence and relaxation, not a crying baby shoved into weary arms. If both parents are working, you have two tired people and a child who may be extra needy of parental attention. Dinner needs to be made, a bath drawn, laundry folded, baby fed, perhaps work from the office attended to. . . . If you like, start screaming here.

Work together to establish a coming-together ritual. On a weekend, sit down together and talk about how you can improve the transition. If you or your mate stays home, you might want to consider these ideas:

Give the working partner an uninterrupted half hour when he or she gets home. In return, you get three hours' alone time on Saturday or Sunday.

The stay-at-home partner might take a walk with your child or find a place to spend the witching hour. In Griffith Park in Los Angeles, a group of parents and children of all ages meets at five o'clock every afternoon in a playground. They can be exhausted and cranky together, and getting the children out-of-doors can distract them from being fussy.

For the partner who comes home: don't make the mistake of rushing past your mate to your baby. Your mate needs to know she is still number one, especially right now. Reassure her, even if it feels obvious and stilted, even if the baby is more compelling right now. You may think she'll be pleased if you pay attention to the baby—true, but only after you pay attention to her.

Consider having a baby-sitter come in one or two days a week late in the afternoon. Look for a preteen who can play with the baby while you remain in the house (preteens cost less). Schedule him or her to remain a half hour after your partner returns home.

Before the witching hour begins, do what you can to relax and unwind. During your baby's last nap of the day, nurture yourself. Listen to a relaxation tape. Exercise. Create a reserve so you can go a little longer.

See But Isn't Self-Nurturing Impossible with Infants and Toddlers?

Talk about how the partner returning home can help. He or she may want "quality time" when the baby is already maxed out; children take in an incredible amount of sensations, and by the end of the day they often have to cry to let off steam. When the partner comes home, adding excitement to an already overstimulated child, it can make the parent who has just gotten the child calmed down feel like a murderous psychopath. In addition, as the child gets older, the parent who comes home is often greeted with such enthusiasm it can make the stay-at-home parent feel awful. Discuss this. What would make you both feel good? What is best for the baby?

When both parents work:

Use the time you commute to unwind. Buy a relaxing tape to listen to in your car or on headphones. Tell yourself, "The workday is done. I did everything I can. I now bring myself fully to my family." If that doesn't appeal, belt back a double martini.

Whoever gets home first or picks the baby up from day care deals with the initial onslaught of chores, getting dinner started, and feeding the baby. This person receives extra time to himself or herself on the weekend. Or switch roles every few weeks. The person who gets home second gets fifteen to thirty minutes alone.

If you have in-home child care, it is worth the extra money to pay your helper to stay an extra half hour. She might be willing to start dinner while you nurse, shower, or play with the baby. Or if this isn't possible, ask her to do simple dinner preparations during nap times.

General witching hour advice:

Connect with each other before you go into survival mode. Stand facing each other, look into each other's eyes, and take three deep breaths together. Acknowledge each other's presence. If you have an older child(ren), include him or her.

Don't take phone calls. Let the machine pick up.

If you can afford it, take-out food is a lifesaver. Whether cooking or not, forget elaborate meals. Take a few minutes together once a week or so to plan a number of simple dishes. Forget variety for a while.

When all hell breaks loose, put on the most relaxing music you have, lie down as a family on the floor or bed, and just give up. Nap, cry together, swear you will never have another child, but stop trying to function. Or sit in a circle (with baby lying down) and massage each other. Or change the energy by going for a walk or a car ride if the weather is bad.

Spray lavender essential oil in the air. Studies have shown this reduces stress.

If your baby or older child has a predictable meltdown time, stop trying to eat dinner during it. Grab some cheese and crackers or have a blender of fruit smoothies ready, and make your own dinner after the baby is in bed. This system can give you uninterrupted time with your mate and older child, if he or she is old enough to wait to eat.

If you do have an older child, enlist him or her as a helper. If you can make your child feel involved, the child will be less likely to add to the tension. Setting the table, rocking the baby in the same room, and washing vegetables are all possibilities.

An early, regular bedtime is the best possible lifesaver for your sanity and your relationship. Yes, this is true even when you both work and feel like you never see the baby. Your baby needs to sleep, and you need to be nourished so you can keep going.

Little Acts of Sacrifice, Empathy, and Appreciation

The ability to enjoy and weather this passage comes in pint-sized packages: the little gestures of love and appreciation that now feel like they take the same energy as planning a surprise vacation to Rio. But you and your lover need these graceful, giving tidbits more than ever. In addition to your favorites, try these ideas:

Tell each other before bed two things you appreciate about each other as parents. Then mention two things that you love about him or her that have nothing to do with parenting.

Treat each other to little indulgences; this can really help to alleviate the stress and boredom of the early weeks. Bring home his favorite glossy magazine, subscribe to a movie channel on cable, send her out alone to browse for CDs, stock up on gourmet snacks, or spring for a nice bottle of wine to sip after your baby's bedtime. Although it is very common to feel stressed out about money right now, it is true that the extra few dollars you spend on Chinese food or videos in the first few weeks won't prevent you from sending your child to college.

Or forget little indulgences and treat yourself to paid help. Everything from taking your car to the car wash to having someone come in and clean can make a huge difference to your sanity.

Institute a code word for when you are about to explode. Use only when absolutely necessary. Your partner is alerted that he or she *must* take the baby and give you a break.

Commit to a regular replenishment night. It doesn't have to be once a week, and it doesn't have to be more than two hours. Discuss the baby only on the ride from home to destination. Once at the restaurant (or park or friend's house), no baby talk. Pick places and activities that were an important part of your life prebaby.

Sex

Couples I spoke with candidly reported not resuming a regular sex life for up to a year after the baby was born. It is not unusual to have sex only once or twice in the first six months. The reasons are multitudinous:

It hurts. Because of hormonal changes, especially if you are nursing, your vagina is drier. A healing episiotomy or sutured tear, as well as the phenomenal changes your vagina goes through during a vaginal delivery, can make sex painful, sometimes for months.

You may fear getting pregnant again. During pregnancy, sex can be great precisely because you don't have to worry about becoming pregnant. With the pain of labor fresh in your mind, you may feel like "nothing is getting in there," as one woman reported.

You don't feel sexy when you have to hold your stomach to keep it from sliding down to your knees.

Who wants to have sex when you could be sleeping?

No time, especially if you have other children.

Leaking breasts. Sex in a puddle of milk somehow loses a little of its charm. (One man in our childbirth class said, "I need to wear a raincoat to bed, she leaks so much.")

Your hormonal balance may leave you uninterested. Masters and Johnson found at three months postpartum women are still experiencing a lower level of sexuality.

You may feel satiated from touching your baby, especially if you are breast-feeding, and not want any other physical contact. When the baby is sleeping, you want yourself back—some psychic and physical autonomy. You don't want to be merging or giving to anyone.

Mothers and fathers don't have sex; normal confusion over your new roles may leave you feeling unsexy.

Resentment—if your partner isn't doing his or her share of child care or housework.

Guilt because you sometimes resent the baby and wish you could have your relationship back the way it was.

Finally, when you do get around to having sex, you may find it unsatisfying. The combination of emotional, physical, and psychological changes can take several months to integrate into your sex life. The first few times you make love, you may feel awkward and stiff, you may not have an orgasm, or it may hurt. It may feel hopeless and very depressing.

The bottom line is: expect a lousy sex life. Expect to have little sex. Who says to have a good relationship you have to make love throughout your life together? What does it matter if there is a temporary lull in the land of heavy breathing?

Pamela Anderson, doctor of Oriental medicine, workshop facilitator, and mother of Samson, believes that if women are truly supported during pregnancy and especially postpartum, they will recover their own energy and sexual selves much faster. She posits the fascinating idea of a woman's partner using touch and sex "to completely serve her needs and heal her after the birth." What if sex (not just intercourse, but cuddling and hugging too) wasn't an issue of "he wants to do it and I don't" or "I'm just too tired"? What if it was rather a way for your partner to support you, actually to give you energy? If your partner can understand the tremendous amount of giving you are doing, as well as your possible need to heal from labor (physically and emotionally), he or she may be able to conceive of sex as a way to help you heal. And of course, someday in the future, you can do the same for him or her—offer touching and sex as a gift.

A gentle way to reintroduce sex is for the new mother to be in complete control. "She can go to whatever limits she wants and quit whenever she feels like it," is what Pamela teaches. "This approach empowers a woman toward sex instead of away from it." This means not that you have to be the initiator, but that you can say, "Please touch me here" and "Please stop. I'm not ready for any more" and "I'm ready for oral sex but not penetration yet."

Ask yourself, "How could my physical relationship with my partner make me feel better during this time?" Think about ways you can nurture yourself and your mate through physical closeness.

Try this cuddling exercise to stay in touch physically: Lie in the spoon position with your partner on the outside. Have your mate gently place his or her hand on an area of your body that needs healing and then concentrate on sending this area healing energy. Your mate matches his or her breathing to yours. Your role is to relax completely. Your partner's role is to send you energy. Breathe together and let go.

If you feel no desire, talk about this with your mate as lovingly and honestly as you can. Make sure he or she understands all the biological reasons you feel this way (you might want to discuss these with your health care provider). See if you and your mate can take the long-term approach by assuring each other that in time you will be more sexually available and giving.

On the other hand, it is important to realize your mate may need you to reassure him that he is still number one, that the baby has not supplanted him in your heart. For men, this reassurance often takes the form of sexual attention. A long, luscious kiss, manual stimulation, or just acknowledging his sexual needs can help him feel loved and connected.

In same-sex partnerships, touch and creative ways to have sex without penetration are probably already a part of your sexual repertoire, so hugging and kissing can psychologically feel like "they count as sex," as Mary, mother of Eli, said. You may feel as if you have more ways to quickly but satisfyingly connect sexually, without squandering sleep time on full-blown, get-out-the-vibrator-and-massage-oil sex.

See Connecting with Your Partner for a further discussion of sexual issues and needs.

Some women report feeling more sexually alive after giving birth than ever before. Go for it! I'm jealous. Enjoy it, but don't worry if your desire waxes and wanes.

Resources:

Becoming Parents: How to Strengthen Your Marriage as Your Family Grows, by Pamela L. Jordan, Scott M. Stanley, Howard J. Markman (Jossey-Bass, 2001). Excellent guidance on a very important issue that we usually ignore.

Fathering Right from the Start: Straight Talk About Pregnancy, Birth and Beyond, by Jack Heinowitz (New World Library, 2001). Straight forward advice for dads, especially good chapter on pregnancy and staying connected.

Fatherneed: Why Father Care Is As Essential As Mother Care for Your Child, by Kyle D. Pruett (Broadway, 2001). A case of involved fathers and clear steps on how to be one.

Great Sex for Moms: Ten Steps to Nurturing Passion While Raising Kids, by Valerie Raskin (New York: Fireside, 2002). Think you are the only one who never wants him to touch your breasts again? Warm, witty, and pratical, Raskin is a M.D. and a mom.

Love Makes a Family: Portraits of Lesbian, Gay, Bisexual, and Transgender Parents and Their Families, by Gigi Kaeser (Photographer) and Peggy Gillespie (University of Massachusetts Press, 1999). Photographs and telling words of children.

The Parent's Tao Te Ching: Ancient Advice for Modern Parents, by William C. Martin (Marlowe & Company, 1999). One of the wisest and most succinct books about parenting.

The Postpartum Husband, by Karen Kleiman (Xlibris, 2001). Help for husbands of women suffering from postpartum depression.

But Isn't Self-Nurturing Impossible with Infants and Toddlers?

You'll Need:

Your journal or paper, and a pen.

From five minutes to an hour or more a day.

When to Do It:

- When your hair is falling out in clumps, you haven't been to the dentist since you were pregnant, and your idea of a sexual fantasy is sleeping next to your mate for eight hours uninterrupted.

- When you don't want to be a mommy anymore, you just want to be alone.

- When you can't even go to the bathroom without a small nose pushed up against the door and the sound of heavy breathing.

What Is It?

Is a self-nurturing mother an oxymoron? Do you want the truth, unvarnished by self-help-book ebullience? Yes, 98 percent of the time. Simply getting enough sleep is often impossible, let alone paddling a canoe, reading a novel, or painting a watercolor. Susan, in her second pregnancy, responded to the question "Have you found any ways to take care of yourself with a newborn or young child?" with "Is this book a comedy?"

Almost every mother struggles for the first few years to maintain her health, let alone a sense of autonomy and balance. Self-nurturing must not become something else you feel you *should* do to be a good mom. This chapter is about addressing some of the internal and social reasons we still needlessly sacrifice ourselves at the altar of mother-hood, and suggestions for surviving.

What to Do:

Why We Feel Guilty and Conflicted

Author and family psychologist John Rosemond writes,

> Taking care of yourself is key to a parent's success in any aspect of child rearing. For example, single parents often ask how they can overcome various disciplinary hurdles with their children. I answer, "Stop paying so much attention to your children, and take better care of yourself."

The current child-rearing dogma is the more attention you pay to your child and the more time you spend with the wee one, the better parent you are. What if that isn't completely true? What if having a life of your own and sometimes putting yourself first is actually better for your child(ren)?

Some mothers voraciously disagree. But even the most ardent proponent of attachment parenting can't disagree with this: you can't give to your child if you don't have anything to give. "Sure, you say. I believe that. But I'm sick of hearing it because it is impossible to nurture myself without feeling conflicted and guilty." I would add, doubly impossible for working and single moms. What to do?

Realize why you feel guilty and conflicted. Self-care smacks of selfishness. It flies in the face of what you have been taught is good mothering. It means you will have to say no to your child, and right now, when your child doesn't understand, saying no for your own sake can be very difficult.

Self-care entails making choices and, once and for all, killing the Perfection Monster. For most mothers (including me), nothing could be harder. Somehow, I don't want to admit I can't cannot write forty hours a week, keep my house immaculate, attend Nicole's wedding in Santa Fe, spend lots of time with Lillian, make passionate love to Chris, and exercise an hour every day (did I leave out maintain a low-fat diet, wear chic, wrinkle-free outfits, and wear lipstick?). How hopeless and ludicrous, but I want to do it all, without help, and be congratulated for it. It is ego gratifying, it means I am indispensable, strong, worthwhile.

It is so hard to choose for fear of failing or disappointing someone else (or my own ridiculous standards). If I admit to myself I'm not capable of doing everything, I'll be worthless. I won't be special. Sound familiar? I hope not. But if it does, know that self-care means you have to set priorities and let things go. No ifs, ands, or buts around it. But it is *tough*.

Melinda Marshall in *Good Enough Mothers* tells the story of Verna, an emergency room nurse with three children, who is struggling to give herself permission to relax.

> Short of doing everything that needs doing, she feels she must "earn" a break and then give herself permission to take it. . . . "I guess it is a question of self-worth," Verna observes. "Women have to believe in the fundamental worth of what they're doing. I'm always asking myself, Is my time spent packing a smiley-face cookie that I decorated myself into Ben's lunch important enough to earn me the right to leave the house and all its obligations? And can I give myself permission to feel unaccountable should the system break down while I'm gone?"

We have to win the right to nurture ourselves. As Avalon, mother of three, put it, "Am I going to lie down and get some sleep, or am I going to scrub your shoes until they're sparkling white?" Because of the Perfection Monster, we never can do enough, earn enough, be sweet enough to deserve time off. But we keep trying to do enough, only to fail because we aren't the Energizer bunny—we can't keep going and going and going. When we fail (by getting sick, making a mistake, or having to say no), we take this not as a warning to slow down but as proof we must try harder, harder, harder to be better, better, better.

Nurturing yourself now takes effort and compromise. "I didn't realize how tense and unhappy I was, how insecure about myself I was beginning to feel. I love Annie, but with all my attention focused on her, I was too wiped out to do anything else. Finally, it dawned on me that it's going to take effort and compromise before I could chase down any time for me again," summarized Penny, mother of six-month-old Annie. Before you became a mother, taking time for yourself probably didn't involve making hard choices. It does now. It will not be easy. Making the effort brings you full circle, back to believing you are worth it and having the courage to spit in the face of the Perfection Monster and to define for yourself what a good mother is.

The final depressing note is the sheer impossibility of finding a moment to yourself. It is simply easier and more comfortable to keep moving, to turn a deaf ear to your needs and emotions, to disconnect from yourself. While in the short term, disconnecting causes minimal damage, the danger comes when it turns into a pattern. You soon lose sight of who you are, which sets in motion a downward spiral of low self-esteem, financial insecurity, and children who view you as a doormat.

If you don't recognize the dictates and pressures against nurturing and valuing yourself, you will not have the courage to keep taking care of yourself. When you sit down to read a book or take Saturday morning for yourself after working during the week, and the internal voice of the "Good Mother" kicks in to tell you how inadequate you are, you will wilt, you will stop, you will give in, and you will go take care of someone else instead. If you know why you are feeling this way, nurturing yourself becomes less daunting.

Practical Ideas for Overcoming Guilt

Nurturing ourselves requires tuning out the clamor of voices and beliefs we have internalized about being a good mother, as well as the racket of "expert" advice. It means we take the time to listen, every day if possible, to our own inner voices, to what we believe is right for us.

See The Spiritual Sustenance of Pregnancy: Strengthening Your Intuition for how-to.

Work on overcoming the voice of the Perfect Mother. When your child is asleep or out with your mate, sit down with your journal and ask yourself, "Where did the voice of this Perfect Mother come from?

See What's Going to
Happen to Me After the
Baby Is Born?: The Myth
of the Perfect Mother *for
help constructing a new
vision of what good
mothering is; and*
Nurturing Yourself During
Pregnancy: Giving Yourself
Permission to Be Good to
Yourself *for how-to
dialogue.*

When does the Perfect Mother criticize me? What does she say?" and "How do I respond to her opinions?" You might try dialoguing with the Perfect Mother. Write down how this internal naysayer berates you and what she believes. You might experiment with drawing a picture of the Perfect Mother.

Realize how callous it can feel to make the hard choice between your needs and your child's. Infants and toddlers can't understand that Mommy needs downtime. Your child may cry and beg you not to leave. This can stop the most determined woman. Try this experiment: Let's say you want to take an hour to paint and listen to music, but you feel too guilty to do so. Don't. Instead, stay with your child but pay attention to how you feel. How much do you enjoy being there? How relaxed and present are you? No judging, just observe. (You might want to write about how you feel, very briefly, in your journal.) Tomorrow, or as soon as possible, take your hour to paint. Then come back to your child and observe how you feel, how patient you are, how present. Prove to yourself that taking care of yourself makes a difference, and use this conviction in the future.

Infancy and toddlerhood are the most time-intensive years of mothering. Even small amounts of time away can be fantastically sustaining, *but only if you give these to yourself often.* You can't go for months without a break and expect a two-hour bath and nap to do the trick. Focus on indulging in slim, tiny, daily ideas. Reading the paper, having an uninterrupted meal, stretching, just being alone takes on a whole new shine. "When you're raising an infant, an hour away seems like half a day," notes Laura, mother of two. However, if you have let your needs slide, don't sabotage yourself by believing that a week's visit to a remote island in the Great Barrier Reef is the only ticket. While that is a fabulous idea, it isn't likely to happen, and while you are waiting, you are going to disintegrate. Start small where you are now.

Stay-at-Home Moms and Working Moms Share the Same Guilt

Stay-at-home moms can feel they don't deserve to spend money on baby-sitters or organize a baby-sitting co-op because they aren't working—and the whole reason they aren't working is to be available to their child(ren). Working moms often feel they must spend every free minute with the baby because they work. Both of these mindsets are dangerous to your well-being!

Stay-at-home moms: value what you are doing, how extraordinarily arduous, complicated, and taxing your role is. You are not less worthwhile or valuable because your job doesn't pay. Deciding you are worth self-care may be the key.

Working moms: you don't have anything to make up for, apologize for, or feel guilty about. You are not doing something bad by working. You must have some time to yourself when you are off. Nurture yourself by killing the Perfection Monster, prioritizing, and simplifying your life.

Making the Time

Perhaps perfection, guilt, or not believing you are worth it is not your problem. But finding any time for yourself when you are not totally wiped out seems about as likely as getting out of the house without spit-up on your shoulder or cereal mashed in your hair.

Adjust your mind to nurturing yourself in bits and pieces, wholeheartedly immersing yourself in the small squirts of time you have. Especially during the first few months, it doesn't help to pine away for uninterrupted hours. Learn to grab what you get and use it, turning off the voice in your head that is worrying about when he will wake up or what Grandma is doing with her.

Put yourself first. When you find yourself with twenty minutes sans children, say firmly to the long list of shoulds clamoring for your attention, "I choose to replenish myself with this time." If the shoulds still make you crazy, split the twenty minutes but take the first ten for you.

Most moms find themselves at loose ends during naps or when their mate takes the child(ren) for a few hours. I would look forward to Lillian's nap with anticipation, only to find myself so hyped up to do something with the time, I would be paralyzed, unsure of whether to exercise, write, read, sit in the sun, return phone calls, or take a shower. . . . When she woke up, it was a queer mixture of relief (now I know what to do with myself), anger at myself (I wasted my free time!), and resentment at Lillian (if I just didn't have a child). When I'm away from her, I miss her and don't know what to do with myself, but when I'm with her, I can't wait for her to go to sleep!

Avoiding this syndrome takes planning ahead. As nap time approaches, decide firmly how you will use your time. Keep a list of simple pleasures handy (see below) to remind you what you enjoy. Post notes around your house: "I choose to use my free time to nurture myself" and "Productivity does not define a good mother" and "Loafing is good for the soul."

Claim a play area so you don't have to waste precious time setting up your space. For example, if working with clay sounds good, keep a card table in the corner with your current project and tools. Or if you exercise at home, keep your weights and videos close by.

Hire someone to do some of your duties. Can't afford it, you say? Pay attention to how you spend money in the next month; just be conscious. How much do you spend on greeting cards? Gifts? Magazines? Just one more adorable outfit for her or one more toy for him? Money tighter than that? What about snacks, soft drinks, ice cream at the mall? Or you think no one you hire will do it as well as you do? Is that the Perfection Monster talking? If help is impossible, organize a chore pool with at least two other parents. Take turns doing errands and grocery shopping for each other; keep photocopies of a master grocery list in the kitchen, then highlight the items you need that week, and write a check when your friend delivers. Do your cleaning together. You get more done and have more fun in less time.

Let your partner be a coparent. *Let* him? It is still common for women not to be completely comfortable, and therefore not completely supportive, of men being equal parents because true coparenting makes us feel like bad mommies, increasing our guilt.

See Receiving the Nurturing You Need from Your Partner Postpartum (and Giving a Little Too): Gatekeeping for more.

Don't make your self-care dependent on others, especially your mate. If he or she won't watch the child(ren) as much as you would like, determine to make the effort to start a baby-sitting co-op. Or locate one other mother you can trade child care with once a week. Or put energy into confronting your partner to do his or her share. Or find trustworthy baby-sitters. To save money, you can hire a younger person to watch the baby with you in the house. You are freed not to fold laundry but to do yoga, watch an old movie *during the day,* or—luxury of luxuries—nap.

Simplify, prioritize, say no. Make this your mantra for the next three to four years.

Accepting Bad Feelings

> Our society simply refuses to know about a mother's experience—how being yoked to a little one all day transforms her. To confess to being in conflict about mothering is tantamount to being a bad person; it violates a taboo; and, worse, it feels like a betrayal of one's child. In an age that regards mothers' negative feelings, even subconscious ones, as potentially toxic to their children, it has become mandatory to enjoy mothering.

So writes Shari Thurer in *The Myths of Motherhood.* When we feel ambivalent about mothering, when we love our children but wish we could turn a switch and deactivate them for a week, we feel even more ambivalent about taking care of ourselves. We feel derelict. Or we don't want to admit our bad feeling because we might start to question whether we are good mothers. We reason that only mothers who are enraptured with their tiny tots at all times deserve an aromatic bubble bath, leg shave, and a glass of ice cold champagne or bubbly apple cider. But what we could say to ourselves about bad feelings is: They are (a) normal and (b) a clear sign we desperately need time out.

In cultures that honor women and mothering, women feel less ambivalence toward their children. Have you ever thought about placing your "bad" feelings in a social context? Have you ever considered that not having enough support makes it tougher? Next time you hate yourself for not loving every minute of mothering, consider how living in this time and place shapes your feelings.

Nurturing yourself before you get totally burned out and frazzled keeps the harpies at bay and your bad feelings in perspective. Before the witching hour, take fifteen minutes to massage your neck and feet and listen to NPR while your baby swings nearby. Before exhaustion has made your complexion gray and your life a blur, take half a day to nap at a friend's apartment (breast-feeding moms can leave one or two expressed bottles behind). If you let yourself get completely depleted, it is almost impossible to recover.

Nurturing Things to Do with or Near Your Child

Take a bath with your child. Light candles, turn on relaxing music, add sweet almond oil to the bathwater. Hold your baby on your chest, lie back, and synchronize your breath.

Hire someone to come to your home and give you a massage during nap time (this works best if your child has a fairly dependable nap time and you won't lie there waiting for her or him to cry).

Find an exercise class or gym that offers baby-sitting. Or find an exercise class for you and the baby; yoga centers are a good possibility.

Invest in (or borrow or ask for them as gifts) good infant-carrying systems, both on the body and in a stroller. A baby carrier (like a sling) can be a lifesaver when you have a wakeful infant. She'll often sleep as long as you wear her. Consider this self-imposed self-nurturing time: plunk yourself down and read, watch a movie, do whatever you really, really want to do (yes, sometimes you can nap this way). If the baby will sleep only while you move, try walking someplace new with her; I favored a historical neighborhood. Take deep breaths. Daydream. Walks with baby can also allow you precious couple time. The baby dozes or stares at the world while you have a chance to connect and get away from the phone and dirty dishes. (This system works only with one infant and only in good weather, unless you are willing to stroll in an indoor mall.)

Get a cordless phone. Keep in touch with adults while nursing, changing diapers, doing laundry.

Make the time you do have alone, like shower time or errands, as nurturing as possible. Light a candle in the shower and play your favorite music. Listen to a book on tape while picking up dry cleaning or commuting to work. Watch an old movie as you fold laundry. Waiting time is "found" time—read a trashy magazine or daydream. Grab those moments and make them nourishing.

Read a poem to your baby during your early morning feeding. Read a novel to your infant; the sound of your voice is what the baby wants. It doesn't matter yet if it is *Charlotte's Web* or *War and Peace*.

Play in nature with your baby. Wade in a stream holding your tot. Plant a garden together (toddlers love to dig in the dirt, and infants love to be out-of-doors). Lie on the Earth naked with your child on your chest. Sniff and pick flowers. Visit the ocean or a lake. Be nurtured by your baby's amazement.

Locate "baby-friendly" places to visit so that you can get out in the world without the added worry of your baby disintegrating into howls while people stab you with murderous stares. Look for shaded outdoor restaurants and loud restaurants, pleasant outdoor shopping malls, hidden parks with water fountains, petting zoos, and baby-loving friends' houses.

Be in the moment with your baby. Stop harassing yourself with everything else you need to get done. Allow yourself to let go and play, to return to that time of innocence, free of responsibility.

See Postbirth Nourishment: Surviving and Thriving: Redefining Time.

Older Children

Accept your children as healers. Children of two years and older love to mommy Mommy. One mother lays a plastic sheet on the floor, gives each of her children a bottle of lotion, and lets them rub her legs and arms, especially her feet. "Kids have a need to give back energy," she notes. Allow your older child to brush your hair, massage your hands, tickle your back, or feed you grapes.

Invest in a Walkman and headphones. When chaos is in full force ("Mommy, mommy"), don your headphones and nurture yourself right in their midst. One mother exercises, another knits, another listens to books on tape; all ignore their children. (Of course, they inform their children clearly and kindly of what they are doing first and make sure their children are within an occasional eye check and in a very safe area of the house.)

Nurturing Things to Do by Yourself

Most new mothers don't have any problem thinking of thousands of wonderful things they could be enjoying. However, as motherhood progresses, you may find yourself having a devastatingly hard time remembering what pleasures you. Try:

Listening to your resentments. Sit down with a piece of paper next time the baby goes to sleep (and your two year old has a play date). Answer the question "I never get time to _____ anymore." Fill in the blank as many times as you can. Do not censor yourself with "But I can't do that now" or "It costs too much." Open your heart to what you've been denying yourself, to a sweeping expanse of nurturing possibilities. Then work on giving yourself small tastes every day.

Answering the question "When _____ happens, I need to nurture myself by _____." When Lillian had colic, I turned to cookies (fistfuls, bags, boxes, heaps, railroad containers of cookies) to soothe my jangled nerves and release tension. Bingeing on sugar made me feel out of control, jittery, and then super guilty when another new mom told me too much sugar in my breast milk made Lillian sweat and her heart race! I found identifying the stresses of mothering and linking these to more self-loving activities helped me to avoid cookie overload (at least some of the time).

Starting a list of miniature pleasures—delights that take only five to twenty minutes. *Write these down;* don't try to keep them in your sleep-deprived head. Buying excellent coffee, wearing something besides grungy sweats, going out to breakfast with baby during nap time (he sleeps peacefully in his car seat while you eat golden waffles smothered in raspberries and read the *New York Times*), sitting still for ten minutes, listening to country music while you play with the baby—these are just a few of the possibilities.

Pondering the question "What activities make me feel centered, authentic, more me?" Act on one idea in the next week.

Things to Remember: Benefits to Your Children

Nurturing yourself benefits your children. Copy this section and give it to your mother or mother-in-law or mothers' group—whoever gives you a hard time about taking time for yourself.

Moms who don't exist to just serve their children—moms who have a life of their own—often find it easier to see their children as separate people rather than as proof of their own adequacy or worth. This is healthy for children because it gives them more space to develop as themselves, free of harsh expectations. It also allows them to learn that the world does not revolve around them, that adults do not exist to satisfy their every whim.

Motherhood does require you to grow and change if you are to do a good job. Your ability to grow into the job is much more likely to happen if you have time away to examine your experiences and understand your feelings. A mom who is constantly on duty is too busy and moving too fast to figure out why she feels rage at her children and how that relates to her own childhood. A mother who never has a break is usually forced to become unconscious to keep from being eaten alive by the intensity of her feelings.

The more you as a mom can love and appreciate yourself, the more your child grows up believing women are worthwhile, exciting people. "By not nurturing myself, I was giving my daughter the message that women are servants who give until they die. When she hears, 'Mommy needs to be by herself now,' she gains a valuable lesson," reports Avalon, a potter and mother of Linnea, Ian, and Somersby.

When you do celebrate and approve of yourself, you are much more capable of celebrating and approving of your child(ren). You have less to prove through your mothering because you are not operating from

But Isn't Self-Nurturing Impossible with Infants and Toddlers?

See What's Going to Happen to Me After the Baby Is Born?: Affirm Your Sense of Self; and Nurturing Yourself During Pregnancy: Postpartum for more ideas.

the belief that you have to do something (like be a perfect mother or win your child's love) to prove your worth. You are able to relax and be present with your child, which in turn allows you to observe and appreciate her or his uniqueness. Children of parents with high self-esteem are much more likely to feel seen and heard for who they are instead of who their parents want them to be.

If you make your child the complete center of your universe, you may have a hard time withdrawing to let the child do his or her own thing. The more you can maintain some sense of personal identity, the easier it is to let go at each stage, from infancy to college to marriage to your child having children of her or his own.

Parenting from a place of self-love allows you to set limits and stick to them, even when your toddler yells, "I hate you." When we need our children to like us so that we can like ourselves, it becomes difficult to deny them anything.

These ideas are not offered to make you say, "Josh, now I must, should, ought to, have to, make myself a priority." They are offered to appease the Perfect Mother—offered so that you can realize your children, as well as you, can benefit greatly from healthy, balanced self-care.

Resources:

Busy but Balanced: Practical and Inspirational Ways to Create a Calmer, Closer Family, by Mimi Doe (Griffin, 2001). An elegant, realistic how-to manual.

Comfort Secrets for Busy Women, by Jennifer Louden (Source Books, 2003). Meet the Comfort Queen.

Times To Treasure Inspiration Cards: 64 Joyful Ideas for Families, by Andrea Alban Gosline (Cedco Publishing, 2001). Lovely, useful ideas on beautiful cards.

Websites:

Getting Things Done
http//www.gettingthingsdone.com

Miracle Organizing
http://www.miracleorganizing.com

The List Organizer
http//www.listorganizer.com

Comfort Queen
http://www.comfortqueen.com

Final Notes

What an act of optimism and faith to bear a child! When you are pregnant, you are on one side of this immense threshold. When you deliver your baby, in the space of a few moments, you jump over the sill and suddenly there you are, you're a mother. Nothing and no one can truly prepare you for this breathtaking passage.

When I gave birth to my daughter, my reaction was, "Oh, that's who was in there." It is shocking to have a *person* come out of your vagina. Personality, soul, spirit, whatever you wish to call it—Lillian was all there the moment we locked eyes. I know my role is to guard her spirit as it unfolds from its seed. She just needs the right conditions to bloom. Becoming a mother is, of course, the same process of unfolding. Everything you need to know you already hold within you. I hope you will have the same patience and reverence for yourself that you do for your child as you grow into your new role.

May your journey into motherhood be held in loving hands of support, framed with time for reflection and pleasure. May you immerse yourself fully in the pools of euphoric joy motherhood bathes you in and traverse wisely but quickly the plunges of despair. May you never forget that the more you are able to give yourself and to receive from others, the more you are able to give your children.

Congratulations.

Creating a lively, grace-filled, flaws-and-all global community of women who are exploring how to creatively, joyfully, fully live their lives is one of the joys of my life. Be part of that community by visiting http://www.comfortqueen.com and by subscribing to my free e-zine newsletter, *The Self-Care Minder.*

You can also reach me at P.O. Box 10065, Bainbridge Island, WA 98110.

Appendix

Herbs, Oils, and Other Natural Comforters

Pregnancy declares almost all drugs off-limits while bringing with it a host of uncomfortable physical symptoms, from hemorrhoids to heartburn. Herbs and essential oils provide safe help, offering one of the best, and often only, ways to get relief.

The recipes here are safe for pregnant and lactating women. However, the responsibility for safety lies with you. You have a unique body, and only you know what works. If in doubt, check with an herbalist or your health care provider. *Beware* of experimenting with herbs and essential oils that are not listed without first checking with a reputable source, such as an experienced herbalist or aromatherapist. Some herbs and essential oils are dangerous during pregnancy.

Ways to Ingest or Apply Herbs and Essential Oils

Herbs can be taken in:

- Capsule form: Potent, quick, tasteless, but also more expensive.

- Infusion: Place the herb(s) in the bottom of a clean mason jar, cover with boiling water, seal, and steep for eight hours; refrigerate to keep. 1 ounce of herbs to 1 pint of water.

- Tea: Most herbs must be steeped for at least ten to twenty minutes; see individual recipes.

- Tincture: You can make your own, but it is fairly involved. Purchase at a health food store or see Resources for how-to books. More potent, easy, and quick, but more expensive; can also be put in a sitz bath.

- Sitz baths: A sitz bath is a shallow bath, not more than one or two inches, designed to keep the water from entering your still-open cervix. Your baby's bathtub, a large aluminum bowl, any shallow container that can support your weight will work. Many women I interviewed stressed what incredible relief baths offered, primarily postnatal. Read, write a letter, meditate, listen to a relaxation tape, or give yourself a facial while you soak your sore perineum in a shallow container for fifteen minutes.

Essential oils can be:

- Mixed in a base oil like almond oil.

- Sprinkled in a warm bath.

- Diffused in a small bowl of hot water or in water over a candle.

- Sprinkled on a cotton ball to sniff.

- Mixed with water and sprayed through a small, glass spray bottle.

Recipes

For general good health, extra calcium, iron, prevention of circulatory problems, and ripening the uterus, make an infusion from:

1/2 ounce red raspberry leaf, 1/2 ounce nettles, 1/2 ounce yellow dock, 1/4 ounce peppermint. Drink one to two glasses a day. Can reheat and serve with honey. Peppermint is for flavor and help with digestion. You can substitute other herbs for flavor. The measurement of the herbs does not have to be exact.

For fatigue try:

Ingesting the entire message of this book: rest, be good to yourself, set priorities, simplify, say no, have fun. Okay, so you have to take care of your toddler, continue to work so you can afford this new creature, and move to a bigger place. How do you keep going when rest isn't possible?

Starting the morning with a cup of spearmint or peppermint tea. No, it doesn't quite jolt the brain cells like a cup of steaming, full-potency Java Joe, but it might bring one eyelid to at least half-mast.

Raspberry leaf: Either in the pregnancy tonic or as an infusion alone. Also instills energy.

Iron: Have your iron checked via a simple finger prick and hemoglobin test.

Acupuncture: From a licensed professional.

For nausea try:

1–2 drops of lemon oil diffused by any means you choose. (Smells are tricky, so if you hate it, chuck it.)

3 drops lavender and 1 drop peppermint essential oil diffused in your room.

2 drops peppermint and 2 drops sandalwood oil on a tissue. Inhale. Or add 3 drops of each to 1 ounce of almond oil and massage into your stomach and chest.

Vitamin B complex, especially B_6, although it shouldn't be taken without other B vitamins, as it can cause you to become deficient in other vitamins and minerals. What you need is a dose of 10 to 20 milligrams of B_6. In severe cases, ask your health care provider about vitamin B shots.

Raspberry leaf: Tea or infusion, depending on which you can stomach. In worst-case scenario, make ice cubes from the infusion and suck on those.

Peppermint: Tea.

Peachleaf: Tea.

Brewer's yeast: Dissolve 2–3 tablespoons of brewer's yeast in juice and drink once. Continue daily with 1 tablespoon in juice.

Ginger: Grate 1 teaspoon fresh ginger root into a cup of boiling water, and let steep for five minutes. Sip slowly.

Dried orange peels: Make a tea of dried slices of grated organic orange peel, steeped for twenty minutes.

Homeopathic remedy: If food makes you ill, try Sepia 6x. If vomiting makes your nausea better, try Nux vomica 6x. If you have a history of anemia, try Lactic acid 6x.

Wild yam root: Make an infusion and sip throughout your day. Or purchase a tincture and take a few drops in water once or twice a day.

Lavender compress: Soak one washcloth in cool water and a few drops lavender essential oil. Soak a second washcloth in warm water and lavender oil. Place the cool cloth on your forehead and the warm on the top of your rib cage.

Sniff peppermint oil.

7 drops lemon oil to 1 ounce almond oil: massage your abdomen with this and inhale deeply.

For mood swings (pre- and postnatal) try:

Motherwort tincture, 5 drops in 4 or 5 ounces of water, no more than three times a day. Combine with a minivacation: take a walk outside, relax your shoulders, do a relaxation exercise.

Raspberry leaf: Infusion for depression. Raspberry leaf alone tastes pretty good, or you can mix in a little peppermint.

Skullcap: Infusion. One cup a day for frayed nerves.

Sniff neroli, lavender, rose, or petitgrain essential oil from a cotton ball or diffuse into your environment.

Homeopathic remedy: 6x to 30x Sepia for depression and inability to think clearly (especially good to use in the first twenty-four hours postnatal); 6x to 30x Pulsatilla for extreme mood swings or a feeling of being "too emotional"; 6x to 30x Cimicifuga for fear.

Massage oil: 15 drops lavender and 5 drops neroli in 3 tablespoons almond oil.

Eat: small, high-protein meals. Snack on almonds. If you can't eat, drink orange juice, milk shakes, or energy drinks to keep your blood sugar regulated.

For heartburn try:

Liquid chlorophyll: 1 teaspoon in an 8-ounce glass of water once a day. Taken daily, chlorophyll may also help your blood to clot, lessening your chance of excessive postpartum bleeding.

Mineral water: Makes you burp.

APPENDIX:
HERBS, OILS, AND
OTHER NATURAL COMFORTERS

See Fear: Controlling Monkey Mind for relaxation ideas.

See It's Not All in Your Head: Surviving the Physical Discomfort of Pregnancy for lots more remedies.

See Tumultuous, Turbulent Feelings for more ideas on dealing with mood swings.

Slippery elm: Lozenges, which are easy to carry around in your purse and tuck in your desk drawer. You can also buy slippery elm dried and mix 1 teaspoon with honey.

Papaya: In tablets (there are many different brands), dried, or fresh. Chew tablets before meals or at the first sign of burning. Eat fresh papaya after meals.

Raw almonds: Chew on a few.

Alfalfa: Capsules.

Apple peels: Chew on a few, organic only.

Massage oil: 1/2 tablespoon sweet almond oil and 2 drops sandalwood oil. Rub gently on your solar plexus.

For varicose veins try:

Butcher's broom: Capsules. (It tastes terrible as a tea.)

Colinsonia: Capsules.

Exercise: Yes, you are tired, cranky, and the last thing you want to do is go for a brisk walk. But even fifteen minutes a day can help. Swimming feels delightful.

Massage oil: To 2 ounces almond oil, add 7 drops lemon and 7 drops cypress oil.

High-potency garlic: Capsules so you won't lose all your friends because you constantly reek.

Extra vitamin E: 600 IU are safe in pregnancy. Check your prenatal vitamins for how much you are getting now, and dose up if more is needed.

Parsley: In salads or as a tea. No more than half a cup a day.

Nettles: Infusion. See general pregnancy recipe above or drink alone.

Bath: Add 3 drops cypress oil and 2 drops lemon to warm, not hot, water.

For hemorrhoids try:

Beet juice: Fresh. Helps cleanse your system, especially your liver.

Witch hazel: Apply directly with a cotton pad. Or make an herbal sitz bath from 1 ounce witch hazel bark, 1 ounce white oak bark, and 1 ounce comfrey. Soak for fifteen minutes three days in a row. Very effective.

White oak bark: Capsules.

Aloe vera gel: Pat on.

Green clay powder: Mix with lecithin oil and pat on. Green clay powder is found in health food stores.

Witch hazel, plantain, and yarrow ointment: check your local health food store for an ointment that contains these elements. Very soothing and effective.

Sitz bath with 2 drops geranium oil and 2 drops cypress oil for ten minutes. Use after fifth month of pregnancy only.

For muscle cramps try:

Calcium with magnesium 1/2 hour before bed: 2 vitamin pills with 800 mg. calcium and 400 mg. magnesium.

Chamomile tea: Contains calcium and can help you sleep.

Stretching before bed: With a flexed foot, not a pointed toe. Also gentle lunges, keeping your heels on the floor. Five minutes of stretching at night makes a difference.

Yoga: Find a prenatal class; the extra training your instructor has gone through will make it much safer and more effective for you.

Heating pad or hot water bottle.

Nettles: Infusion. See general pregnancy recipe or drink alone.

Massage oil: To 1 ounce almond oil add 4 drops lavender and 4 drops geranium oil. To be used after fifth month of pregnancy. Mix well and have your partner or yourself massage your legs before bed.

Breath: When the cramp occurs, breathe into the pain. Think of this as practice for labor. Remind yourself the cramp will pass.

For headaches try:

Raw almonds: Chew at the first sign.

Ice pack: Where the pain originates from, alternate with a hot pack.

Skullcap: Tincture: 3–8 drops in 6 ounces of water. Can make you drowsy.

Lavender oil: 1 drop on each temple.

Vitamin E: 600 IU are safe in pregnancy. Check your prenatal vitamins for how much you are getting now, and take more if needed.

Peppermint: Soak a washcloth in cool water and a few drops peppermint essential oil. Apply to your forehead.

Eating: Try more protein and less sugar.

Sleep!

For insomnia try:

Skullcap tincture: 30 drops in 6 ounces of water 1/2 hour before bed.

Bath: Warm water with 3 drops lavender and 3 drops mandarin oil. Also try diffusing lavender, neroli, sandalwood, or ylang-ylang oil in your bedroom. Frankincense oil sprinkled on a tissue near your pillow or otherwise diffused in your bedroom is supposed to help ease nightmares.

Calcium with magnesium: 2 pills 1/2 hour before bed.

Chamomile: 2 capsules or a cup of infusion, taken 1/2 hour before bed.

Tea: Lavender, lemon balm, linden, and chamomile. Take an equal pinch of each and steep in a covered pot for twenty minutes. If too flowery, use less lavender.

Milk: Put a cup of warm milk in your blender with one banana and a tablespoon of honey. Sprinkle with cinnamon.

For healing of genital herpes or to prevent an outbreak try:

Pau d' arco: A Brazilian herb. Capsules. Follow package instructions.

Lysine: An amino acid. Capsules.

Vitamin E oil: Apply directly to the sores.

Milk of magnesia: Let the fluid settle, then apply the white particles (for pain relief only).

Hair dryer: Use a low setting to promote healing.

Calendula: Cream found in health food stores and sometimes well-stocked drugstores. Also good for certain types of diaper rash.

Food: Eat fish, chicken, beef, cheese, brewer's yeast, soybeans, eggs, milk, spinach, asparagus, and green beans because they contain more Lysine.

Avoid nuts (including peanut butter and coconut), brown rice, whole wheat bread, oatmeal, raisins, and chocolate (oh no, not chocolate!).

Vitamin C: 2000 mg. are safe during pregnancy. Check your prenatal vitamins to see how much you are taking now. If you find yourself having loose stools, decrease the amount.

For congestion try:

Eucalyptus, pine, or tea tree oils: 2 drops of one or the other in a bowl of hot water. Cover your head with a towel and inhale the steam for 5 minutes. Also, diffusing a few drops of these oils around your environment helps.

For healing your perineum after birth try:

Vitamin E oil: After tear is well closed. Apply as frequently as you like. Be sure to keep the area extra clean because the oil attracts dirt.

Sitz bath: 2 drops lavender oil and 2 drops cypress oil. Once a day if you have stitches, up to three times if you don't. Fifteen minutes a sitting.

Another sitz bath: 1/2 ounce comfrey root, 1/2 ounce white oak bark, 1/2 ounce witch hazel bark, 1/2 ounce ginger root, 1/2 ounce golden seal. If you don't have all of these herbs, use whatever ones you have. Steep herbs in boiled water for twenty minutes, then soak your perineum for twenty minutes. The sitz bath should be as warm as you can tolerate.

Ice packs: Thirty minutes every one to two hours.

Witch hazel: Apply it with a gauze pad. Feels great if the witch hazel is chilled.

For sore nipples try:

Vitamin E oil: Rub it on after nursing and wipe off before.

Seeing a lactation specialist. You might need to work on nipple placement.

No soap: Splash your nipples with warm water and air dry.

For engorged breasts try:

Hot ginger compresses: Grate fresh ginger root onto a washcloth, soak in hot water, and hold on your breast until it cools.

Hot showers.

Have your baby feed in small, frequent feedings and from both sides.

For breast infections:

Hot compresses: Before nursing, then a cold compress afterward.

Goldenseal: Mix a small amount (approximately 1/2 teaspoon) of the goldenseal powder in 1 teaspoon or so of castor oil. Smear all over your breast. Apply a wet, warm washcloth, then wrap with plastic wrap, then cover entire poultice with a heating pad. Hold for ten to twenty minutes.

Potato peels: Cover the lumps in your breast with potato peels. Cover with plastic wrap, and hold for twenty to thirty minutes.

Nurse: A lot! Change positions with each nursing, if possible alternating between cross cradle (the standard position), football hold, and lying down.

Massage: Toward your nipple, especially while nursing.

For postnatal "adjustment" try:

Baths! Warm, not hot. Add 5 drops of clary sage and 3 drops ylang-ylang oil. Or 2 drops neroli, 2 drops petitgrain, and 2 drops orange essential oil. Or add the same amounts to 2 1/2 tablespoons of sweet almond oil and have someone massage you. (This recipe is Allison England's special pick-me-up from her book *Aromatherapy for Mother and Baby*.)

Showers! If you don't have time to bathe or can't yet because your cervix isn't closed, sprinkle 2 to 3 drops of your favorite essential oil on a sponge and brush over your body after you've washed.

Lemon balm: An infusion tastes good especially with honey. One to two cups a day.

Blessed thistle leaves: Tincture works best. Up to 80 drops a day.

See Postbirth Nourishment: Surviving the Emotions.

From *After the Baby's Birth* by Robin Lim, a general postpartum tonic: A generous pinch of comfrey, false unicorn, licorice root, red raspberry leaves, and shepherd's purse to 1 gallon boiling water. Steep for fifteen minutes or longer. Sip throughout the day.